THE INVISIBLE FORCE

Traditional Magnetic Therapy
A Consensus of Practical Opinion

Fred Rinker C.M.T.A.

The Invisible Force

1997
Published by
Mason Service Publishing
C.P. 27106
London, Ontario
Canada N5X 3X5
Phone (519) 660-0491

The original art in this book
is the work of artist
Frank Northgrave
Elliot Lake, Ontario, Canada

Manufactured and printed in Canada

ISBN 0-9681900-0-6

Acknowledgments

THE POWER THAT MADE THE BODY,

HEALS THE BODY,

IT HAPPENS NO OTHER WAY.

B. J. Palmer

I would like to acknowledge the help of all those who contributed to this work; my son Mark, my daughter Lynda and my wife Frances. They not only provided advice, support and guidance but tolerated my obsession with completing this project. I would like to apologize to the rest of my family especially my son Chris and my 6 grandchildren for the lack of time to be with them more over the last several months.

A special thank you to Dr. Ken Wiancko, Bob Grace and Gale Weisenbarger, all of whom offered invaluable support and direction.

I wish to commend Canadian artist Frank Northgrave for his insightful cover design and fine line drawings.

CONTENTS

Introduction

The Invisible Force

Life developed under the influence of the earth's geomagnetic field. We are surrounded by a sea of magnetism. The human body, its individual organs and each of the millions of cells making up the organs and the body bathed by this sea are magnetically charged. Cell regulation, tissue function and life itself are controlled by internal electromagnetic currents. In disease states, these electromagnetic potentials are altered but fortunately can be favourably influenced by the external application of magnetics.

Conventional medicine has long opposed alternative treatment techniques. Many of these techniques encompass age old methods blending body and mind, science and experience, traditional and cross-cultural diagnosis and treatment. A recent New England Journal of Medicine study reported 1/3 of American patients chose an alternative therapist over conventional medical treatment and 2/3 of patients had visited a complementary therapist over the last year. No estimates were given as to the numbers that had elected to take responsibility for their own health care using self-administered alternative therapies.

Over the last 90 years illness as cancer, heart disease, arthritis, hypertension, infections, chronic fatigue, headaches, digestive problems and numerous aches and pains have become such an integral part of our lives that they are accepted as normal. Death and disability from these diseases has not been appreciably changed by all our modern, expensive and potentially lethal therapeutic practices. It's been reported that between 60,000 and 140,000 people die in the USA each year from drug reactions prescribed as "standard" therapy by establishment physicians. Many of these toxi- chemical killing drugs are prescribed for non-life threatening conditions.

Magnets have been used for healing since antiquity. Their benefits have been recorded in ancient Egyptian, Greek, Chinese and other writings. Until recently, although the health improving potential of magnet therapy was well documented, scientific explanation of magnetic action was not available. Dedicated researchers and the introduction of the space age have contributed greatly to the understanding of the physiology of magnetism in health and healing.
Many health problems, once diagnosed by the medical profession, can be treated effectively and safely by the patient using magnets without resorting to potentially dangerous drugs. The use of magnets is simple and the benefits can be immense.

Magnets aren't magic. Their use isn't quackery. Magnets have been scientifically proven to be able to assist the body regain its self-healing electromagnetic balance naturally.

Ken Wianeko, M.D., F.R.C.S.(C), F.A.C.S.
Diplomate of the American Board of Chelation Therapy

Preface

My initial interest in magnets developed from a chance discussion with a friend. He later found, and gave me a book called <u>The Anatomy of Biomagnetism,</u> written by Albert Roy Davis Ph.D. Shortly after reading the book I visited Dr. Davis' research center in Florida and met with his associate Walter Rawls. Their pioneering work with magnets was fascinating and prompted them to co-author four books on the subject. I later became acquainted with Dr. Richard Broeringmeyer, an author, lecturer and authority on magnetic therapy. His newsletters, books and manuals were of special interest as he had worked closely with Davis and Rawls.

The study of magnets and their various applications has remained a major focus of interest. For 20 years I have researched and studied the available literature on the subject. I have talked and corresponded with many of the pioneers in this field, including Dr. William Philpott of the USA, and others from North America, Europe, India and Australia. I was certified as a magnetic therapist through the Magnetic Therapist's Association of Australia and was later named Canada's Honourary Representative to the International Council of Magnetic Therapists.

The principal books and literature available on this subject are listed in the bibliography. A study of this literature reveals serious contradictions, in that opposite polarities are recommended for treating the same ailment. When one determines how each writer identifies polarity, then examines the recommended treatments, all fundamentally agree with one another. It is reassuring to see the same basic conclusion when the correction is done for polarity identification. This common understanding of polarity effects, is a major factor in confirming the validity of magnetic therapy treatment.

The contradictions as mentioned are disturbing and offer a major stumbling block for those wishing to study and fully understand this valuable treatment method. In addition there is considerable misunderstanding and misinformation with regard to the gauss strengths of magnetic materials and products.

Another area of concern is the apprehension of PMF, or Pulsed Magnetic Field therapy. This may be the result of negative publicity regarding electromagnetic pollution.

Magnetic therapy and other natural therapies are often condemned by conventional medicine because of the lack of published double blind studies. The use of magnets and magnetic therapies are not considered patentable, which detracts large agencies and companies with research funds. Because of this, clinical trials have rarely been conducted in North America. This area of study is much more advanced in Eastern Bloc countries, where drug therapy is scarce and unaffordable. Europeans have also been more vigorous in the research and acceptance of magnetic therapy.

If the simple application of a magnet can control a typical pain condition, it eliminates the need for normal drug-based pain medication. One can assume this fact has not gone unnoticed by the established pharmaceutical and medical supply industries, which may feel obliged to discourage and discredit alternative therapies.

As our population ages, magnetic therapy will have an important contribution to make as an alternative treatment for chronic pain. This is evident by the vast acceptance it has already received at the grass roots level. It is an indisputable fact that health care costs are spiraling out of control. The demand for inexpensive methods of health care is obvious.

Magnetic therapy is a non-invasive treatment method with a very high success rate. There have been no problems with side effects and contra-indications are well known. Anecdotal evidence, and scientific verification becomes stronger and more valid as results are recorded regarding the effectiveness of specific treatments. Magnetic therapy has much to offer in both the prevention and treatment of chronic ailments.

My main purpose in writing this book is to harmonize the various opinions and establish a consensus with regard to treatment methods and polarity. My secondary purpose is to further the study and understanding of magnetic therapies.

This book offers a consensus of opinion on magnetic therapy, with consideration given to the products and equipment generally available. It is written to be easily understood by practitioners and their patients.

CHAPTER 1

Magnetic Therapy Yesterday and Today

The earliest recorded use of magnets dates to 800 BC. Physicians in ancient Greece, Egypt, India and China described and practiced magnetic therapy and it was mentioned in the writings of Homer, Plato, and Aristotle.

Aesculapius is considered the founder of the healing arts. All American physicians swear on his name when taking the Hippocratic Oath. In his book <u>Magnetic Therapy</u>, Abbot George Burke explains that the ancient writings tell us Aesculapius healed mostly through the application of magnetism.

Magnetic therapy is no longer ancient history nor a mysterious force. Science has established that magnetic energy passes through all material and affects all living things. Magnetic fields surround the earth and protect all living things from harmful radiation. They also influence mans behaviour, mental function and physical energy.

Magnetism is a basic natural force of the universe. It is the basis for new discoveries in all fields of applied science. This includes electronics, chemistry and physics. The commercial and industrial applications of magnetic energy are as common as the electric motor in every machine. Magnetism plays a major role in everyday functions, from simple domestic appliances to the most advanced scientific instruments.

Modern medicine is beginning to realize the potential value of using magnetic energy in the treatment of physical and mental disorders. In 1989, the FDA and the University of Tulsa jointly sponsored a conference on emerging electromagnetic medical technology that attracted researchers, physicians and specialists from around the world.

Research for space exploration has produced important information on the human response to magnetic fields and pulsing magnetic frequencies. NASA discovered that magnetic field generators installed in manned space ships were essential in maintaining bone density and normal health for the early astronauts. They found that specific magnetic fields and frequencies produced certain biological responses. The Earth's natural pulsing frequency of 7.96 Hz (cycles per second) reduces stress and encourages relaxation and sleep. Sound, restful sleep is essential in achieving top physical and mental performance.

The most significant use of magnetic energy in conventional medicine is through magnetic resonance imaging (MRI). A sophisticated diagnostic tool, MRI employs the different effects of the two poles on the hydrogen factor in human tissue to create an image otherwise unavailable. The MRI system detects and details soft tissue and is important in detailing the brain and detecting tumors. Teeth and bones that contain little water do not appear on an MRI image. Other approved devices include EEG, MEG and SQUID diagnostic equipment, which can also detect and record important electromagnetic information.

The FDA has approved PMF (Pulsed Magnetic Field) treatment for non-union bone fractures. The treatment device is available by prescription only and is custom made for each patient, therefore, it is an extremely costly application procedure.

A set of bar magnets applied to either side of a fracture provides a similar effect as does the application of PMF treatment using a standard miniature device available off the shelf.

Other applications using magnetic and electromagnetic energy are infrared heat therapy equipment, ultraviolet purification systems, magnetic hearing aids, and homeopathic, colour and light therapies. Kinesiology test equipment and magnetic probes which remove metal particles from the eyes, nose and ears can also be included.

While some diseases and disorders respond best to orthodox medicine, conventional medicine and alternative therapies can work in harmony. Natural alternatives are generally safer with fewer side effects and should be considered whenever possible.

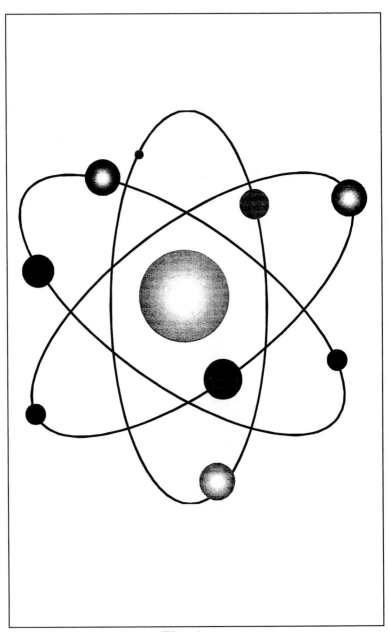

The Atom

CHAPTER 2

Expert Opinions

In his book, <u>The Body Electric</u>, Dr. Robert Becker observed that an injury site registers South-positive immediately. It changes to North-negative during the healing process, indicating that a North-negative field promotes healing.

Dr. William Philpott explains the pH factor and the calcium factor in his book, <u>Cancer The Magnetic/Oxygen Answer</u>.

- Reduced ionized calcium plays a major role as a common denominator in degenerative disease, in addition to acidosis. Reduced ionized calcium is not necessarily related to a lack of calcium in the diet. It is more likely related to reactions to environmental pollutants that cause an acid response in the body. He states that calcium and other minerals can only remain in a soluble state in the presence of an alkaline medium. In acid mediums they become insoluble.
- Negative magnetic fields oxygenate and alkalize by aiding the body's defense against bacteria, fungi, and parasites, all of which thrive in an acid medium. In degenerative diseases, calcium is found deposited around inflamed joints, bruised areas on the heel, and in bones and kidney stones. Infections occur because they function well in an acidic, oxygen deficient state.
- A negative magnetic field combats inflammation and infection and enables the body to resolve troublesome calcium and mineral deposits.
- A negative magnetic field is effective in relieving pain due to its oxygenation and alkalinizing action.
- A negative magnetic field enhances deep restorative sleep. The pineal gland produces melatonin in the presence of a negative magnetic field.

- Oxygen and water are paramagnetic and can carry a magnetic field to all parts of the body through blood circulation.

Dr. Philpott states that negative magnetic energy is capable of filling indented skin where a tumor has been. He also reports that no scar tissue will form where a cancerous tumor is neutralized by North pole magnetic energy. The same magnetic energy field eliminates scar tissue formation when a cut heals.

Dr. Philpott's findings support Dr. J. Bischko's studies at the Ludwig Boltzmann Clinic in Vienna, Austria. Dr. Bischko used bipolar magnetic pads.

Dr. Philpott postulates that when a negative magnetic field is applied to a diseased internal organ, such as the liver, a three month application of negative magnetic energy may be required to cure the disease. An additional three month application may be required to repair the organ. His advice is to ensure that the magnet being used is larger than the lesion being treated and that sustained treatment with negative energy from a permanent magnet be applied.

Dr. K. Nakagawa's study, <u>Magnetic Field Deficiency Syndrome</u>, states the human body is under the influence of the earth's magnetic field and is keeping some sort of a balanced relationship with it. However, under modern day living conditions, the effect of this magnetic field has decreased. Consequently, in some situations we can assume that this lack of magnetism has caused some abnormalities. By applying a magnetic field on the human body to supplement this deficiency, such abnormal conditions can be improved. In other words, there is a direct relationship between the decrease in the earth's magnetic field on the human body and the improvement of abnormal conditions by the application of magnetic fields.

NASA reported the early astronauts suffered from a magnetic field deficiency while orbiting in space away from the earth's magnetic field. This caused some serious medical problems including a rapid loss in bone density. This deficiency was corrected by providing an artificial magnetic field in the spacecraft.

Research by Dr. J. Bischko and Dr. Peter Kokoshinegg at the Ludwig Boltzmann Acupuncture Institute, and the Institute of Biophysics and Ray-Research in Vienna, Austria, indicated the following; Scar tissue breaks down and new skin forms when an alternating field magnetic pad is applied.

TDK Industries of Japan carried out three important studies where magnetic necklaces were tested to find their effectiveness in treating stiff shoulders. The conclusion was that magnetic necklaces effectively reduced discomfort in 81.1% to 96.3% of subjects. No noticeable side effects were found in respect to the clinical examination results. (Magnetic necklaces produce alternating pole energy)

Dr. Ken Wiancko MD, wrote an article (Health Naturally, April 1996) that stated: "Though they seem magical in their ability to heal, magnets are not magic. Their function is very simple. Magnetotherapy helps the body to regain its self-healing electromagnetic balance naturally because each organ and each cell of every organ in the body is influenced by electromagnetism. Cell regulation, tissue function and life are controlled by electromagnetic currents.

In Dr. Nakagawa's classic study, Magnetic Deficiency Syndrome, he outlined that lack of magnetism may cause stress, mental disorders, headaches, arthritis, muscle pain, osteoporosis, chronic fatigue, allergies, insomnia, in-flammation, circulatory problems, bowel disorders and other degenerative problems afflicting people today. Universal cure-all? In the search for a universal cure-all, none fit the description nearly as well as magnetic energy therapy. The application of magnets has given proven pain relief in seven out of ten users, as good as or better than "orthodox" medicine. Magnetotherapy is far less expensive and lacks the dangerous side effects often associated with prescription drugs. However, proper advice and care should be taken when using strong and large magnets about the head. Treatment with magnets is not addictive and does not interfere with other therapies, but should not be used if a pacemaker or defibrillator is worn.

Researchers have stated that magnetic field therapy rebalances altered metabolic functions that cause pain, edema (tissue swelling), excess acid in the tissues, and lack of oxygen in the cells, thereby initiating tissue healing and pain relief. Skin calcification, the cause of skin aging and wrinkles, disappears. Joint mobility increases and muscles become more flexible. Digestion improves, prostates shrink and kidneys eliminate body wastes more effectively. Mental function increases, energy levels go up and sleep is better. Tests have even shown that organisms placed under a magnetic field live longer.

Because it potentates the body's free radical scavenger and antioxidant system, magnetotherapy is reported to be valuable in counteracting degenerative processes causing heart and circulatory disease, arthritis and auto-immune illness, as well as neuro-degenerative and allergic afflictions. Drinking magnetic water is said to impart many similar benefits. Wearing back, neck or joint supports with permanent magnets imbedded in the material often relieves painful conditions.

Treatment of discomfort from strains and arthritis with low frequency, pulsating magnetic fields created by tiny portable devices may be as effective as larger ultrasound units.

Stress causes hundreds of diseases but can be tempered by using magnets day or night. Nighttime magnetic field therapy has a calming and sleep inducing effect on the brain and body due to stimulating production of melatonin, an anti-stressful, anti-aging and anti-infectious hormone. Sleeping on magnetic mattress pads can improve the quality of sleep and eliminate morning stiffness.

Magnetotherapy may often be used as a first line treatment for pain and to promote healing, not to suggest that there is no place for standard prescription drugs. Many distressing conditions yield to magnetics, but if magnets don't help, it's important that you visit your doctor."

Dr. Ulrich Warnke: Magnetic energy has a beneficial effect on blood circulation, lymph flow, hormone production, nerves and muscles.

Dr. Evelyne Holzapfel: The application of a magnetic field has the virtues of simplicity, freedom from danger and low cost.

Dr. Madeleine F. Barnothy: The magnetic field will develop into a powerful new analytic and therapeutic tool of medicine.

Dr. Kenneth S. McLean: This treatment (magnetic therapy) is a godsend. It's good for almost everything.

Dr. Louis Donnet MD: Besides being easy, efficient and inexpensive, magnetic therapy offers a total guarantee of safety.

Dr. Ralph U. Sierra: We now stand on the verge of a great new age in magnetic science and its applications -- a tool that has been provided by Mother Nature herself.

Neville S. Bengali MD: The astounding results obtained through magnet therapy give it a place of considerable importance in the field of therapeutics.

Dr. J.B. Baron MD: This is a revolution in the therapy of muscle injuries, joint pain, and posture problems. We have treated 4,000 patients with whiplash injuries by means of the magnet and cured 80 percent of them.

The First Congress in Magnetotherapy organized by the Coghill Research Laboratories was held at the Royal Society of Medicine in London, England in May 1996. The proceedings introduced over 50 studies and research reports on magnetic therapies, the majority of which were very positive. For example three doctors from Croatia published an outstanding report outlining the treatment of 1261 patients in a rehabilitation hospital using PMF therapy.

Eastern Bloc countries have traditionally researched magnetic therapy much more vigorously than the West. Many of the studies presented at the First Congress in Magnetotherapy originated in countries where magnetic therapy was seen as an economical option to drug therapy.

CHAPTER 3

Magnetic Therapy - How it Works

Magnetic therapy utilizes the natural energies of magnetism that are important to human existence and overall health. Human beings possess complex bio-electromagnetic systems, while all electro-systems also contain magnetic fields. A magnetic field provides a natural way to assist the body as it passes through all tissues and cells

The outer surface of each nerve cell carries a positive charge, while the interior of the cell carries a negative charge. In the case of pain, the positively charged cell membrane is supplied with more potassium by the blood, thereby increasing the positive charge. As a result, a powerful current flows through the cerebral neurons, which register the event as pain. If the site of the pain is exposed to a magnetic field, the different charges are neutralized, the current flow declines and eventually ceases altogether. In most cases, the pain is alleviated.

Magnetism is very effective for healing and restoring the natural balance of the body. This helps to bring a normal charge back to each body cell by increasing cellular oxygen and restoring pH balance. The cells then become well. The use of an external magnetic source helps the body in the healing process, alleviating the need to deplete its own energy resources.

Several studies on the effects of magnetic fields reveal that blood flow increases under the influence of magnetic fields. This fact can be proven with infrared thermography which uses different colours in the image to define different skin temperatures. In 1983, Dr. Ulrich Warnke conducted tests on both humans and horses, revealing that electromagnetic fields increased blood flow by dilating the blood vessels.

This was observed in the thermographs within 2 minutes. Other studies using the same technique indicate similar results using bipolar magnetic pads.

The Theoretical Significance Of Left And Right Electron Spin In The Human Energy System, Encyclopedia Britannica 15th edition Vol. 15 (1986). Proteins pp 859-880, Carbohydrates pp 881-890, Lipids pp 891-896.

"A static magnetic field is an energy field by virtue of the movement of electrons. The negative magnetic pole moves (spins) electrons to the left and the positive magnetic field moves electrons to the right. Electron movement is the essence of energy. Light also is an energy by virtue of its movement of electrons. Polarized light can move electrons either to the left or right depending on the refractory ability of the substance through which it is going.

Oxygen and water are paramagnetic and can be magnetized as either positive or negative. Magnetized oxygen, or water, will behave like a static magnetic field being either positive or negative, depending on the magnetic field to which it has been exposed.

It is important to understand that the magnetic field that spins electrons to the left supports the body's energy oxidation-reduction process. It seems evident that this negative magnetic field supplies the energy for the enzyme function, the reversal of acids, hydrogen peroxide, and oxygen free radicals, thus releasing molecular oxygen from these products which can be used in the oxidation process of energy production in the human body.

The human body requires an alkaline medium because an acid medium cannot maintain oxygen and is toxic to the human body. A negative magnetic field supports the body's alkalinity and high need for oxidation capacity for energy production.

Magnetic North pole oxygen or water supports human physiology. Oxidation provides energy for reversal and reduction of end-products (free radicals, hydrogen peroxide, and acids) and aids in maintaining the necessary alkaline pH."

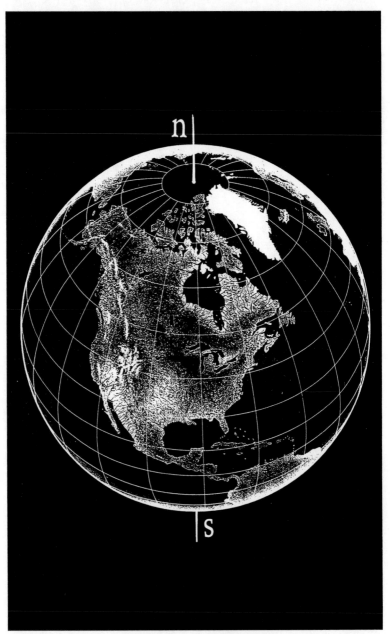

The Earth And Its Poles

CHAPTER 4

Polarity

The sources of information on polarity are geographically diverse. One must carefully interpret each author's definition of polarity when studying the literature. While some authors use the correct application with regard to their particular understanding, they identify polarity incorrectly. This means that they identify polarity opposite to its biomagnetic designation. Their information is perplexing to many who have attempted to study and understand the application of magnetic therapy.

The problem began when science and industry established a standard method to identify the polarity of magnets. They marked North on the end of a magnet that pointed to the earth's North pole, and South on the end that pointed to the earth's South pole. This designation is incorrect, but is used to this day by all manufacturers and industrial suppliers of magnets. It was an innocent mistake because no one understood the different effects of the two poles. They did not give consideration to the following basic rule:

Opposite poles attract, and like poles repel

The earth's North pole attracts the South pole of a magnet.
The earth's South pole attracts the North pole of a magnet.

The recommended magnetic applications in this book conform with the biomagnetic polarity designations established by Dr. Albert Roy Davis and Walter Rawls, which have been proven in thousands of tests and experiments.

The Davis-Rawls Biomagnetic identification of polarity:

- **North Pole or Negative polarity** The side or end of a magnet causing the same reaction as the earth's North pole when using a compass. Since opposites attract, this is also known as the South seeking pole.

- **South Pole or Positive polarity** The side or end of a magnet causing the same reaction as the earth's South pole when using a compass. Since opposites attract, this is also known as the North seeking pole.

Bipolar or Alternating polarity Describes a magnet or magnetic field that provides a pattern of alternating North-negative and South-positive impulses. This effect can be produced with permanent magnets used in an alternating (bipolar) pole pattern or with PMF (pulsed magnetic fields) in an oscillating wave pattern.

To date, alternating magnetic fields from both permanent magnets and electromagnetic equipment have received the most interest from a research standpoint.

TDK Industries sponsored an important study with regard to the effects of alternating pole magnetic necklaces on out-patients at the orthopedic department of Japan's Kohnnodia National Hospital. The results indicated a high percentage of improvement.

The effects of PMF therapy are recorded in many studies. Dr. Benjamin Lau of the Department of Microbiology, School of Medicine, Loma Linda University in California conducted a significant study on the effects of low frequency electromagnetic fields on blood circulation. Dr. Lau concluded that low frequency, low intensity alternating electromagnetic energy may be beneficial in clinical

conditions where an increase of tissue oxygen is thera-
peutically desirable.

Note - Do not confuse passive magnetic fields and PMF
magnetic fields used in magnetic and electromagnetic therapy
with electromagnetic fields produced by EMF high tension
electricity, TV screens, computer monitors, and electrical
appliances.

Permanent magnets do not produce frequencies, the Earth is
the lone exception. Pulsed Magnetic Field therapy equipment
transforms alternating current to direct current, which
produces pulsed magnetic fields in set frequencies. Battery
powered devices also use direct current to produce alternating frequencies.

The information in this book adheres to the following
definitions:

North Pole = **Negative polarity**

South Pole = **Positive polarity**

Both Poles = **Bipolar** = North and South Poles applied
simultaneously; also called alternating poles

PMF = Pulsed magnetic fields in an alternating North-South
wave pattern

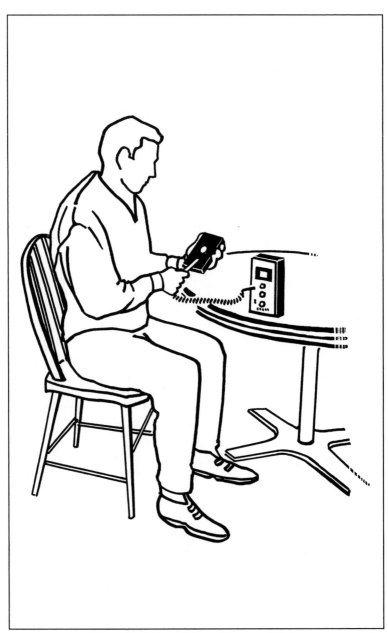

Measuring with a Gauss Meter

CHAPTER 5

Gauss and Gauss Ratings

The following description and explanation of gauss was developed from an original article by Gale Weisenbarger, a knowledgeable expert in this field. Mr. Weisenbarger was concerned about the misinformation he found in the marketplace.

He refers to, The Permanent Magnet Design and Application Handbook, written by Lester Moskowitz, to provide the following definitions and explanations.

What is Gauss

Gauss is the cgs unit of magnetic induction. Magnetic induction is the flux per unit area, measured at right angles to the direction of the flux.

Important facts about Gauss

Manufacturer's Gauss rating This refers to the strength properties of a specific magnetic material which is used to compare and rate different types of magnetic material.

When magnetic products are described in terms of the manufacturer's Gauss rating of the material they are made from, many incorrectly believe that these magnetic products have been measured and that this "Gauss rating" describes the actual magnetic strength of the product.

Gauss is not a standard number indicating the strength of every magnet made from the same material.

Each magnet made from the same material will have a different Gauss reading based on size, weight and shape.

Magnets used for biomagnetic purposes are described as "open-circuit" magnets because they do not have supplemental ferromagnetic parts to provide a complete path for the magnetic energy. Any type of basic unfinished magnet falls into this category, including magnets used in mattresses, body wraps, jewelry, magnetic disks and blocks.

Gauss Ratings (byAuthor)

The following provides factual information on the actual gauss properties of different magnets and magnetic products. Gauss must be measured with a gauss meter not a magnetometer. A Gauss meter is a calibrated precision instrument used to measure lines of magnetic flux at a specific point on a magnet. This reading provides little information about the total energy of the magnet being tested or how far the energy will project from its surface. To produce the following results I used a Gauss meter with a flat probe supplied by AZ Industries. This company is a well known manufacturer of quality magnetic instrumentation.

Each magnetic object was measured for the following qualities:

1. The actual Gauss of each magnetic object measured at the highest reading point.

2. The distance in inches from each magnetic object where the magnetic field is reduced to 2 Gauss.

3. The distance in inches from the magnetic object where it begins to produce an effect on a compass.

The Gauss measurements recorded indicate the following conclusions:

1. Manufacturer's Gauss rating of magnetic materials does not directly relate to:
- The actual Gauss readings recorded on the surface of individual magnetic objects

2. Actual Gauss readings of magnetic materials are directly related to:
- The type and grade of the magnetic material
- The polarity orientation of the magnetic material
- The size and shape of the magnetic object

Gauss Readings from Selected Magnets

1. Highest Gauss measured on magnet's surface
2. The 2 Gauss point measured from the magnet's surface.
3. The Compass detection point in inches from the magnet

Description					1.	2.	3.

Ceramic Magnets (3,950 - 4,000 Gauss)

Description					1.	2.	3.
1 Disk	3/4"	x	3/16"		600	3"	7"
2 Disks stacked	3/4"	x	3/16"		900	3 1/2"	11"5
5 Disks stacked	3/4"	x	3/16"		1,050	4"	13"
9 Disks stacked	3/4"	x	3/16"		1,150	4 1/2"	18"
18 Disks stacked	3/4"	x	3/16"		1,160	5"	36"
Disk	1"	x	5/16"		600	3 1/2"	9"
Disk	1 1/2"	x	1/2		700	12"	20"
Disk	2"	x	1/2"		700	14"	26"
Rectangle	1/2" x 3/8"	x	3/16"		500	2"	5"
Rectangle	1 3/4" x 7/8"	x	3/8"		600	5"	15"
Rectangle	2" x 1"	x	1/2"		600	6"	15"
Rectangle	2" x 5"	x	1/2"		700	13"	32"
Rectangle	2" x 5"	x	3/4"		800	14"	40
Rectangle	4" x 6"	x	1/2"		800	13"	60"
Rectangle	4" x 6"	x	1"		980	18"	72"

Description				1.	2.	3

Neodymium Magnetic Material (12,300 Gauss)

Disk	3/8"	x	1/10"	1,700	2"	5"
Disk	1"	x	3/8"	2,000	7"	20"

Magnetic Rubber - High Intensity (2,500 Gauss)

Strip	2"	x	1/16"	x	6"	100	5"	11"
Strip	3"	x	1/8"	x	6"	200	6"	12"
Strip	3"	x	1/4"	x	6"	300	8"	20"

Magnetic Rubber - Bipolar

.030" thick gold back (diamond)	180	3/8"	1 1/2"
.060" thick gold back (diamond)	260	3/8"	3"
.045" thick silver back (parallel)	120	3/8"	3"

Individual magnetic devices (as described)

Magnetty 1,000 - (bipolar) 5/32"	240	1/2"	2"
Magnetty 6,000 - 1/8"	1,200	1"	2 1/2"
Magnetty 9,000 - 5/32"	1,300	1"	3"
Expansion bracelet (ceramic)	500	1 1/2"	4"
Expansion bracelet (neodymium)	1,700	2"	5"
Bracelet with 1/2" magnetic balls	300	2"	3"
Ear studs 7/16" dome shape	600	2"	5"
Necklace black onyx bipolar	300	1"	5"
Necklace black onyx	400	1 1/2"	6"
Magnetic insoles 1/8" all North	25	4"	12"
Magnetic insoles 1/8" (bipolar spaced 1/5")	150	1/2"	2"
Magnetic insoles 1/8" (bipolar spaced 3/8")	200	1/2"	3"
Magnetic insoles 3/16" (bipolar diamond)	170	1/2"	2"

CHAPTER 6

Magnetic Materials

The Materials

Basic treatment magnets fall into several categories. The older type of conventional iron magnet is seldom used in North America however it is still popular in some Asian countries. This type of magnet is generally low powered and loses its strength quickly.

The common types of magnets in general use are as follows:

Alnico is a high energy alloy made of aluminum, nickel, iron, cobalt, and copper. Alnico is not often used in magnetic therapy due to its high cost compared to ceramic.

Ceramic magnets are man-made. They are produced from fired clay as well as barium ferrite, a type of iron in very fine powder form. The material is mixed with water into a matrix, then heated to a molten state at approximately 1,800 degrees F. The molten material is then poured into molds to cool and be processed in a high powered electrical magnetizer, which magnetizes the material. This process produces a fine permanent magnet that will retain its magnetic field for many years. One must handle this type of magnet with care since it is quite brittle and can be easily broken. Ceramic magnets are usually coated with epoxy or plastic for protection. Several grades are available, with Ceramic #5 and Ceramic #8 being the most common grades used for therapeutic purposes.

- Ceramic #5 magnetic material has a manufacturer's rating of 3,950 gauss.
- Ceramic #8 magnetic material has a manufacturer's rating of 4,000 gauss.

Ceramic block magnets are used for direct application in magnetic therapy. They vary from small domino sizes to various bar and slab shapes up to 4" x 6" x 1". Circular disks from 3/4" to 1" in diameter are used in a wide variety of magnetic wraps and appliances. Similar magnets are used in magnetic mattress pads and pillows.

Samarium-Cobalt magnets are also used, though they are not as common or as popular as ceramic or neodymium materials. Various grades have manufacturer's ratings from 8,700 to 11,000 gauss.

Neodymium is a high priced magnetic material made from neodymium, iron and boron. This mixture of rare earths and metal produces a very high strength material. The most common grades used by therapists are:
- Neodymium # 27 magnetic material with a manufacturer's rating of 10,800 gauss.
- Neodymium # 35 magnetic material with a manufacturer's rating of 12,300 gauss.

Neodymium is available in disk shapes and small blocks. The material must be carefully coated and protected as the iron content is subject to rust. If exposed to moisture the magnet could be seriously damaged.

Flexible Magnetic Rubber - Mono Pole This material is available in 2 and 3 inch strips with thicknesses of 1/8 inch and 1/4 inch. The magnetic field is oriented through the thickness, providing North pole on one side and South pole on the other. High intensity magnetic rubber has a manufacturer's rating of 2,400 gauss.

Flexible Magnets - Bipolar This material is available in several pole alignments. These include parallel lines, squares, circles and diamond patterns. Alternating North-South pole patterns produce a good magnetic field at the surface. The opposite poles in the patterns are self-inducing (attract each other). This prevents the magnetic field from projecting more than 2 to 3 inches.

The different pole patterns have little effect on magnetic field strength. Gauss strength directly relates to the thickness of the material and the quality and amount of iron powder in the rubber. Depending on these factors, the various products available on the market have manufacturer's ratings of 400 to 700 Gauss. The actual Gauss measurements vary widely depending on the thickness and the spacing of the poles. The table on page 34 details the actual measurements of some of the more common items available.

Mini Magnets - Spot Magnets - Magnettys These are small magnets, approximately 1/8" in diameter that are made with ceramic, samarium-cobalt and neodymium materials. Lower strength ceramic units are bipolar while higher strength units are single pole. The magnets are pre-pasted on adhesive strips, ready to apply and are available in several grades. The single pole magnets are reversible allowing either pole to be used as required. The bipolar magnetty 1,000 provides 100 gauss while single pole units of grade 2,500 provide 200 gauss. Grade 6,000 provides 1,200 gauss and grade 9,000 provides 1,300 gauss. An acupuncture point finder is helpful in locating treatment points.

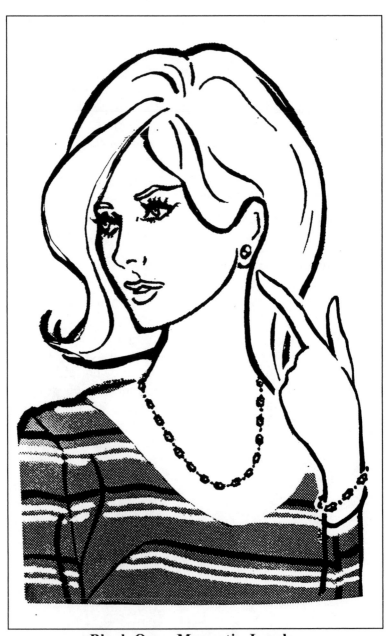

Black Onyx Magnetic Jewelry

CHAPTER 7

Magnetic Products and Properties

Magnetic Jewelry Finger rings, wrist bracelets, expansion wrist bands of various strengths, magnetic bracelets, ear studs and a wide variety of necklaces are all available. Magnetic jewelry generally offers an alternating pole effect though some items such as expansion bands are available in an all North pattern. Neodymium magnetic pendants are commonly used to stimulate the heart and thymus.

Magnetic Mattress Pads Models made in North America usually present the North pole side toward the user. These are often reversible. Some models made in Asia present the South pole while others utilize an alternating pole pattern. Ceramic disk magnets are the standard component in typical mattress pads. These disks vary in diameter from 3/4" to 1" and are usually 3/16" thick. The spacing varies, but is usually 3 to 4 inches on center. High strength models feature domino sized ceramic block magnets placed closely together. Magnetic mattress pads are available in all standard bed sizes. Some high priced models have the magnets built into an elaborate mattress system.

An alternative method provides a high strength sleeping system using 4" x 6" ceramic block magnets. Ten or fifteen magnets are placed in a pattern with the North side up between the box spring and the mattress. This provides a high powered magnetic bed. Magnets placed this far down will eliminate any effect of opposite pole feed.

Magnetic Pillows These are usually made with magnets embedded in a foam pillow. Some models provide pockets that allow larger magnets to be positioned on the underside. It is important to ensure that the magnets presented to the head are North pole. In addition to promoting deep restorative sleep, magnetic pillows are helpful to those with upper shoulder and neck problems.

Magnetic Pillow Inserts An insert can be slipped into the pillow case allowing one to turn their pillow into a magnetic pillow. Placing the North pole side up at the bottom of the pillow will eliminate the opposite pole effect.

Magnetic Body Wraps The wraps are made to fit specific body areas including the instep, ankle, calf, knee, thigh, back, shoulders, neck, head, elbow and wrist. They usually provide an elasticized material to hold the magnets and a velcro closure to keep them in place. North pole and alternating pole wraps are both available. Some models are made in the form of elasticized sleeves.

Magnetic Pads Several types are available. Pads similar to small mattress pads have many applications as body wraps and can also be used as seats. Others in this category are small flexible pads made with neodymium magnets embedded in layers of foam.

Rubber Magnets Flat magnetic pads of flexible rubber material are available in two basic types:

- Strips of rubber magnetic material, often described as plastiform attach to the body with an elastic bandage or wrap and allow application of either North or South pole energy. Some body wraps use this material as the magnetic element.
- Alternating pole magnetic pads are available in various sizes, shapes and pole patterns. They provide both pole (bipolar) energy and can be used alone or applied with tape or elastic bandages. Various magnetic products are made using alternating pole inserts as the magnetic element.

Magnetic Insoles and Shoe Inserts Several types are available. The basic insoles are made of plastic with small magnets in various locations. Higher quality types use flexible rubber magnets with various coverings to provide durability and comfort. The alternating pole pattern is generally used. This provides a strong magnetic field to all areas of the foot producing increased circulation and pain control. Magnetic insoles are used in reflexology and energy balancing. Insoles are also available in North pole orientation. These have a lower magnetic field strength, but are useful in the treatment of foot infections.

Magnetic Face Mask The stimulating effect of magnetic energy benefits wrinkled areas of the face and restores a youthful appearance to the skin. This application also offers relief to acne sufferers as the North pole energy produces an alkalizing effect which helps eliminate infection and skin eruptions.

Magnetic Pendants Usually made from neodymium. The pendants are used over the sternum to provide oxygenation to the blood. In his work with cancer patients and magnets, Dr. Goesta Wollin used neodymium pendants to provide magnetic stimulation to the thymus gland.

Note: Magnetic products made in Asia usually have all South pole or alternating pole patterns. You need to know the polarity of your product to use it correctly. A small compass can be used to check any item you plan to use. A magnet's North pole side will attract the compass needle that points to the Earth's North pole. A magnet's South pole side will attract the compass needle that points to the Earth's South pole. If you wish to apply North pole energy you can often simply use the reverse side of a South pole product.

Common Questions Asked

How do magnetic fields interact?
Les Adam of AZ Industries is an acknowledged expert in the field of advanced magnetic application. He offers an interesting illustration on how magnetic fields interact.

- Picture the magnetic energy field surrounding a magnet as a bubble similar to an air bubble. As two magnets of the same polarity are moved toward each other, the energy bubbles begin to change shape as they come in contact with each other. The closer the magnets get to each other, the more distorted their energy bubbles become. A magnetic energy field, like an air bubble, will interact and change shape as a similar field comes in contact.

What is opposite pole feed?

- Often called South pole feed, this term describes the natural effect of the opposite pole magnetic field appearing between magnets in a pattern using one polarity. This opposite pole magnetic field can be measured with a gauss meter. For instance, an item such as a mattress pad made with magnets in an all North pole pattern, will produce a small South pole effect through the spaces between the magnets. This opposite pole energy will be about 5% of the main magnetic field. This small opposite pole effect has not produced any known problem from the millions of mattress pads being used that are made this way. For anyone concerned, this effect can be eliminated with any standard mattress pad by positioning the magnetic layer a few inches below the sleeping surface.

Do permanent magnets block electromagnetic pollution?

- No. Claims that wearing magnetic pendants or other devices made of permanent magnets will absorb or block electromagnetic waves are incorrect. There is no published research that substantiates this claim.

Do magnets help with electromagnetic pollution?

- North-negative   magnetic energy from a pendant or magnetic disk will increase negative ions that may help offset the effect of positive ions absorbed from electromagnetic pollution.

How important are the pole patterns of a bipolar magnet?

- Alternating pole magnets are usually flexible rubber pads with a magnetized iron content. The magnetic energy is produced from alternating North - South poles on the face of the magnet. This layout produces a high strength magnetic field considering the thickness of the magnet.
- The majority of published research has used parallel line pole patterns. This research indicates exceptional results in both human and animal studies. The principle reason offered for the positive results is the Hall Effect. Other pole patterns that have been developed include concentric rings, checkerboard squares, and diamond pattern designs. These seem to perform as well as the parallel line pattern. Pole patterns do not appear to be an important factor.

What is meant by the Hall Effect?

- The Hall Effect is the generation of an electric potential perpendicular to both an electric current flowing along a thin conducting material and an external magnetic field applied at right angles to the current upon application of the magnetic field. [After Edwin H. Hall (1855-1938)].
- The Hall Effect explains the effect of polarity alignment placed at right angles to the blood flow. Since blood flows in all directions in the body, any alternating pole alignment will produce the same general effect.

Are bipolar magnetic fields harmful?

Based on the vast amount of research indicating the absence of side effects and in consideration of the obvious contra-indications, the answer is NO.

Is North pole energy harmful?

- The literature, in particular that originating in North America, explains North-Negative polarity as the contracting, healing, alkalizing polarity. This effect in the long term would not benefit anyone in a weakened condition or bedridden for 24 hours a day. One should spend no more than 8 to 10 hours a day on a North pole magnetic mattress. Condition caused by excessive alkalinity would not benefit from prolonged North pole exposure.

Is South pole energy harmful?

- Eastern Bloc Countries have recently translated and published many important studies on magnetic therapies. Many of these studies utilize permanent magnets in addition to electromagnetic devices. There is no distinction given to the application of either polarity. These studies have generally produced very positive results.

- There are several books on this subject by Indian authors who use the industrial designation of polarity that is opposite to the biomagnetic definition. When their recommendations are reversed the literature makes sense and the polarity effects agree. They utilize the benefits of the South pole effect to much greater extent than has been practiced in North America.

- The studies published in Japan pay little attention to polarity. Magnetic products made in Japan utilize all South pole or alternating North-South patterns of polarity.

- French literature supports the Davis-Rawls definition of polarity and recommends using the South pole application when a stimulating effect is required.

- Chinese literature describes an energy system called Chi which uses both polarities to restore the body to a balanced harmonious state. The terms "Yin" and "Yang" describe opposites, such as negative and positive polarities.

- The vast majority of scientific research on this subject is based on the use of electromagnetic devices that produce alternating magnetic fields.
- The potential side effects of North and South pole energy were not mentioned in studies by the World Health Organization and The American Food and Drug Administration on potential harmful effects of magnetic fields.
- There seems to be no particular hazard from either of the Earth's magnetic poles when one considers the health of living creatures in both hemispheres.
- South pole energy exists in each magnet as well as in each cell of the human body.

The answer to whether South pole energy is harmful or not weighs heavily in favour of using South pole magnetic fields when it is appropriate. South pole energy is important. When used correctly and with balance it can provide many benefits.

Note: When applying South pole energy, one needs to consider the effect of using high strength South pole fields for prolonged periods and in any situation where stimulation could be harmful.

Are electromagnetic fields from PMF therapy harmful?
Other than the stated contra-indications, it can be said that PMF therapy is safe in comparison with other types of therapy, i.e. drugs and electrotherapy.

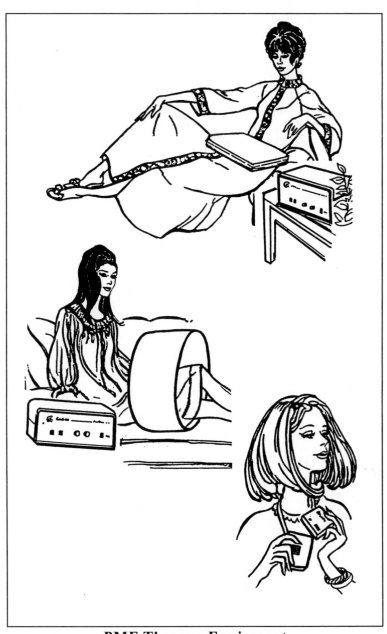

PMF Therapy Equipment

CHAPTER 8

PMF Pulsed Magnetic Field Therapy

PMF devices produce pulses of alternating magnetic fields. The biologically compatible, magnetic energy subjects nerve and cell tissue to changing electrical potentials, which may induce a temporary analgesic effect and promote healing of damaged tissue.

PMF devices utilize 120 volts of electricity (240 volt in some countries). This power is transformed to produce an alternating pulse at various frequencies. Portable models are powered with either 3 or 9-volt batteries.

Magnetic therapy devices were developed in North America during the last century. In some instances responsible practitioners produced great results but controversy developed when scam artists began to sell ineffective devices at inflated prices. This gave magnetic therapy a poor reputation with conventional medicine that exists to this day.

After World War II many new advances were made by researchers in eastern Europe, particularly Romania and Russia, in the application of magnetic fields. In the late 1960's electromagnetic therapy was introduced and further developed in Germany. Dr. Wolfgang Ludwig and Dr. Hans Brugemann were prominent in the early research. The German company, Elec GmBH, was one of the early commercial producers of electromagnetic therapy devices. Their product line, which included equipment for both human and veterinarian application, was used in the early 1970's. By 1986, Elec claimed that over 2,000,000 patients worldwide had been treated with several thousand devices in hospitals, clinics and universities. Their equipment was being used by researchers at a number of major universities including The University of Loma Linda in California, Texas

A&M University, the Universities of Modena and Bologna in Italy and the University of Saarbrucken in Germany.

The German Elec device has been copied and cloned in many countries. Though the original concept has changed little, Australians may now be at the forefront of advancing and refining this technology. PMF therapy equipment is currently produced in many countries.

Many professional sports teams utilize electromagnetic therapy equipment. Other specialized equipment is used in the race horse industry and by equestrians to rehabilitate injured horses. It is claimed that both human and equine athletes return to active status in half the normal time when using PMF therapy.

Miniature battery powered PMF therapy units are produced in Austria, Canada and Australia. These devices produce low energy magnetic fields in frequencies ranging from .5 Hz (one pulse every 2 seconds) to 50 Hz (50 pulses per second). The Canadian device uses an advanced antenna technology developed by Dr. W. Ludwig of Germany, which has 7 variable switches which enable it to produce over 100 different frequencies. A new product from Australia has 3 frequency selections, using a different approach to the wave form. It uses extremely short oscillating pulses between 4 and 16 Hz. It is said to identify more at the atom level in the molecule rather than at the cellular or tissue levels.

The Biological Effect of Pulsed Magnetic Fields

The effects of pulsed magnetic fields are proven and have been illustrated using infrared thermography. The thermographic pictures show a temperature increase due to an increase in blood circulation caused by the application of pulsed magnetic fields.

The basic cell of an organism can be influenced by a pulsing magnetic field of certain frequency and intensity. It is recognized that in certain diseases, the resting and threshold potential of cells within the organism differ from the norm, thus impairing the function of the cell. Pulsed magnetic fields completely penetrate through every cell.

The improvement of oxygen transport and oxygen saturation is due to the magnetic influences on hemoglobin at extremely low frequencies. At the cellular level the effects are increased oxygen diffusion in the cells, increased cell metabolism and mineral exchange.

A pulsed magnetic field is clinically established to have analgesic, antinflammatory, and antiodemic effects. It improves circulation, accelerates tissue regeneration and provides a regulatory effect on the nervous system.

Pulsating magnetic fields are known to produce the following effects among others:

- Relief of pain and inflammation
- Stimulation of tissue
- Increased circulation
- Rehabilitation of tissue
- Increased relaxation (low frequencies)
- Increased bowel movements (high frequencies)

These effects have helped in treating the following ailments:

- Diseases of the support and locomotory system, in particular rheumatic and arthritic disorders
- Sports injuries such as bruises, pulled or torn ligaments and muscles, tennis elbow
- Delayed wound healing
- Non union fractures
- Headache and migraine

- Heart and circulatory diseases, circulatory disturbances
- Metabolic disorders
- Neuralgia
- Bronchitis and sinusitis, acute and chronic
- Skin ulcers

Contra-indications with PMF therapy:
>(especially with higher frequencies and high power)

- Pregnancy
- Pacemakers
- Hemorrhage
- Viral infections (high frequencies)
- Juvenile Diabetes
- Menstruation (high frequencies)
- Hyperthyroidism
- Active tuberculosis
- Acute viral conditions
- Malignancies (high frequencies)
- Neurological diseases with seizure
- Severe atherosclerosis

CHAPTER 9

The Magnetic Effect

- A magnet or an electromagnet produces an energy field

- Each pole of a magnet produces a different effect

North-Negative	South-Positive
Has a counter-clockwise rotation	Has a clockwise rotation
Inhibits	Excites
Relieves pain	Increases pain
Reduces inflammation	Increases inflammation
Produces an alkaline effect	Produces an acid effect
Reduces symptoms	Intensifies symptoms
Fights infections	Promotes microorganisms
Supports healing	Inhibits healing
Reduces fluid retention	Increases fluid retention
Increases cellular oxygen	Decreases tissue oxygen
Encourages deep restorative sleep	Stimulates wakefulness
Produces a bright mental effect	Has an overactive effect
Reduces fatty deposits	Encourages fatty deposits
Establishes healing polarity	Polarity of an injury site
Stimulates melatonin production	Stimulates body function
Normalizes natural alkaline pH	

Supplementing the earth's magnetic field by sleeping on a North pole magnetic mattress or by wearing magnetic jewelry and other magnetic devices helps restore the natural magnetic field. Wearing a negative magnet over the heart provides the body with magnetic energy through blood circulation.

PMF -- Alternating Magnetic Fields

Pulsed magnetic fields produced by PMF treatment devices are characterized by low frequency, low power, micro oscillating direct current. The following effects have been recorded:
(Hz = cycles per second)

- .5 Hz   Produces a sedating effect and pain relief
- .5 to 4 Hz   Stimulates the auto-immune system
- 5 Hz   Increases DNA synthesis
- Under 10 Hz   Vaso-constrictive, reduces blood flow
                 and inflammation
- 12 to 15 Hz   Vaso-dilative, increases blood flow,
                 oxygen and nutrients
- 18 Hz   Increases metabolic rate

The Safety of Magnetic Fields

The arrival of magnetic resonance imaging (MRI) has led to extensive testing to determine toxicity and safety of magnetic fields associated with MRI equipment. The FDA has classified magnetic field exposure, as "not essentially harmful".

The World Health Organization's study of magnetic fields, Environmental Health Criteria 69 MAGNETIC FIELDS, published in 1987 states (p. 20), "It can be concluded that available knowledge indicates the absence of any adverse effects on human health due to exposure to static magnetic fields up to 2 Tesla (20,000 Gauss)".

The static magnetic field from a permanent magnet is an energy field. This can be illustrated by observing the two different effects that a magnet has on the electrons which sustain the image on a black and white TV set or computer monitor.*

- When the biomagnetic North-negative pole is brought slowly up to the screen one can observe the image on the screen rotate to the left (counter clockwise).
- When the biomagnetic South-positive pole is brought slowly up to the screen one can observe the image on the screen rotate to the right (clockwise).

This simple test not only indicates the effect of a passive magnetic field but also illustrates the basic difference between the two polarities.

* Caution: Do not carry out this experiment using a color monitor. The magnetic field will demagnetize the screen. This can be reversed by a TV repair person with the proper equipment.

Side Effects

No adverse side effects have been observed with negative magnetic energy, the healing energy of the Earth. However, if pain or pressure increases with the application, one should first try to move the magnet. If the problem persists, then the magnet should be removed. Pain can be caused by pressure from fluid buildup. Since negative magnetic energy pulls additional fluid into an enclosed area, pain can increase if direct application is made to an area already full of fluid with no drainage capacity. In this instance moving the magnet above, below or beside the painful site will pull fluid away from the affected area and relieve the pain.

Precautions

- A magnetic mattress should not be used 24 hours a day. It should be used no more than 8 to 10 hours per day because some body functions may be suppressed. Other magnetic wraps or pads may be used throughout the day on painful areas.

- Do not use magnetic energy on the abdomen for 60 to 90 minutes following a meal.
- Do not use South-positive magnetic energy on any area of the body that may be affected by stimulation, such as an infection, inflammation or a tumor.
- Do not place a large ceramic block or high energy magnet near the head for prolonged periods.
- When using magnetic therapy in the treatment of asthma and emphysema, begin cautiously as coughing or choking may result from congestion breaking up quickly.
- Persons on medication may develop symptoms of over-medication when using prescription drugs in conjunction with magnetic therapies. The magnetic effect will reduce stress and inflammation as toxins are released and metabolism improves. Drugs can become more effective and may need to be reduced or discontinued as the body's chemistry changes. Consult your health care provider if symptoms occur.
- Do not use magnets during pregnancy.
- Do not use magnets or PMF therapy if using a pacemaker.

Magnetic therapy should not be considered a panacea but should be utilized as part of an overall treatment strategy.

CHAPTER 10

Therapeutic Guide

At the onset of any disease or new symptom, it is recommended to consult a health care professional. Magnets and magnetic therapy are able to mask pain. It is paramount that one establish the reason for pain before starting any treatment. When the specific medical condition is identified, select the method of treatment to use, whether it be conventional, alternative or both.

Definitions:

North Pole = Negative Energy

South Pole = Positive Energy

Both Poles (Bipolar) = North and South poles used together

Alternating Poles = North and South poles used in sequence.

PMF = Pulsed Magnetic Fields

The following treatment recommendations are based on a consensus of opinion from all available sources.

Abscess (boil)
Use South pole to bring abscess to a head, then North pole to dry up the infection. Drink North pole water and use it to wash the affected area.

Acidity
Apply a North pole magnet to the pain focus. Drink North pole water. PMF therapy is an option with this ailment.

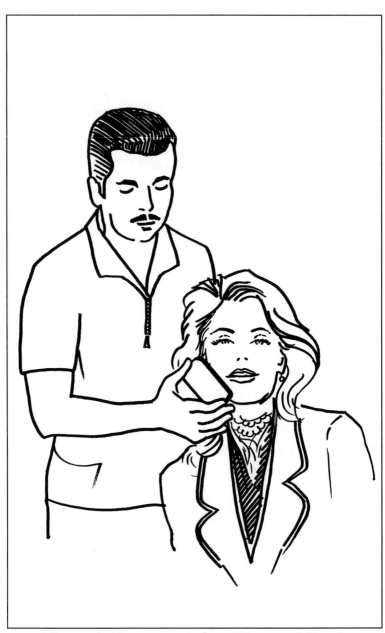

Magnetic Treatment of an Ulcerated Tooth

Acne
Use a North pole magnetic face mask. Drink North pole water. **See Skin**

Adynamia (weakness)
Use an alternating North-South magnetic wrist band. Sleep on the South pole side of magnetic mattress to expose the spine to South pole energy. Turn the mattress over and sleep on the North side at least once a week. Use a North pole magnetic pillow. Drink water magnetized by both poles. PMF therapy is an option with this ailment.

Age (old age ailments)
PMF therapy should be considered as a treatment method.

Allergies
PMF therapy is an option with this ailment.

Alopecia - See Hair loss

Amenorrhea (suppressed menses)
Use the South pole of a rubber strip magnet on the pubic region and the sacral area. Apply for 30 to 60 minutes twice daily. Rebalance with North pole.

Angina
A professional diagnosis is essential. Use magnetic therapy as a supplement to conventional treatment. Wear a small North pole magnet in the breast pocket or attached to clothing over the heart area. Discontinue use immediately if discomfort is experienced. Drink North pole water daily. Do not use magnets with a pacemaker.

Anxiety - Refer to Stress

Anemia

Drink magnetic water exposed to both poles. PMF therapy is an option with this ailment.

Anorexia

Use the South pole of a ceramic block magnet over the upper abdomen or the spine in line with the navel. Rebalance spending equal time with North pole. Wear a South pole magnetic wrist band on the left wrist. Drink water magnetized by both poles.

Apoplexy - See Stroke

Appendicitis

A professional diagnosis is essential. Acute appendicular pain may require hospitalization. Use magnetic therapy as a supplement to conventional treatment. Alternative treatments for chronic appendicitis would include the application of the North pole side of a rubber strip magnet to the lower right abdomen.

Arthritis (osteo)

A professional diagnosis is essential. Use magnetic therapy as a supplement to conventional treatment. Apply North pole magnetic energy using a magnetic mattress. For pain control apply North pole magnets over the region with magnetic products specifically made for use on wrists, hands, elbows, shoulders, backs, knees, ankles and feet. Alternating pole magnetic pads will help alleviate pain from tense muscles and tendons caused by arthritic pain. PMF therapy is an option with this ailment. Drink North pole magnetic water daily.

Arthritis (Rheumatoid) - See Auto-immune disorders

Arteriosclerosis

A professional diagnosis is essential. Use magnetic therapy as a supplement to conventional treatment.

Arteriosclerosis (legs)

Either North or South pole energy may be applied as conditions dictate.

- South pole will vasodilate the artery wall, allowing the artery to open as far as possible, increasing circulation to the legs and feet. However, the South pole while increasing circulation, may also increase pain. The South pole should not be applied if high blood pressure or varicose veins are a factor.
- North pole will sedate the pain. If high blood pressure is a factor use North pole energy only.

Please note: The choice of which pole to use only applies to the extremities such as the legs. Use North pole energy only in the heart area. A small North pole magnet may be worn in the breast pocket or bra, but do not use magnets with a pacemaker or defibrillator. Drink magnetic water made with both poles.

Arrhythmia

A professional diagnosis is essential. Consider magnetic therapy a supplement to conventional treatment. PMF treatment may be beneficial.

Arthrosis

Stimulate the area with PMF treatment.

Asthma

Expose the chest to both poles. Place one large ceramic block magnet to the front and one to the back in such a way that they are opposite one another. PMF therapy is an option with this ailment. Begin cautiously as congestion broken up too quickly may cause increased coughing. Drink water magnetized with both poles.

Auto-immune disorders

There are many diseases in this category including; Lupus, Rheumatoid Arthritis, Multiple Sclerosis, Chronic Fatigue Syndrome, Crohn's disease, AIDS and Cancer.

A professional diagnosis is essential. Use magnetic therapy as a supplement to conventional treatment. Use a high strength North pole magnetic mattress and pillow. A magnetic pendant may be worn over the sternum to stimulate the thymus gland. Drink North pole water daily.

Atrophy
Apply a South pole or an alternating rubber magnet to the affected muscles. Drink water magnetized with both poles daily.

Backache (injury)
Use a North pole magnetic pad or mattress overlay. Lower backache can be effectively treated with a North pole magnet. Use a North pole on any new injury initially. A recurring injury (chronic) may also respond to South pole stimulation once healing has begun. Chronic kidney pain can be treated with a large North pole ceramic magnet. If discomfort persists, see your health care professional. Drink water magnetized with both poles daily.

Back Pain (Arthritis, Sciatica Lumbago, Scoliosis, Whiplash and Coccyx pain)
Consult a Chiropractor or Osteopath to determine the cause. North pole magnets are recommended for pain control. Alternating pole magnetic pads are recommended if the muscles are affected. Use a North pole magnetic mattress and pillow. Magnetic belts using North pole or alternating polarity may also be effective. Flexible magnetic strips and flat ceramic blocks may be used while lying or sitting. Drink North pole magnetic water.

Bed Sores (pressure sores)
Sleep on a North pole mattress pad. The foam type is best. Wash the area frequently with North pole water.

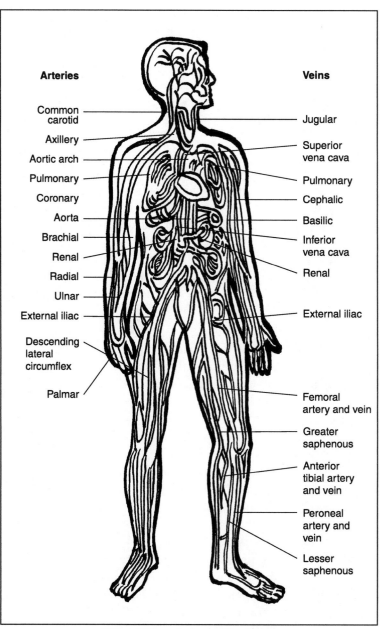

Arteries

Common carotid
Axillery
Aortic arch
Pulmonary
Coronary
Aorta
Brachial
Renal
Radial
Ulnar
External iliac
Descending lateral circumflex
Palmar

Veins

Jugular
Superior vena cava
Pulmonary
Cephalic
Basilic
Inferior vena cava
Renal
External iliac
Femoral artery and vein
Greater saphenous
Anterior tibial artery and vein
Peroneal artery and vein
Lesser saphenous

The Circulatory System

Bee Stings
Apply North pole magnets as soon as possible to reduce swelling and alleviate pain. Wash the area with North pole water.

Bell's Palsy
Use the South pole of a medium sized ceramic or flexible magnet on the affected facial muscles. Apply on the facial nerve just behind the ear on the affected side.

Biliousness
Apply a North pole magnet to the upper right abdomen. Drink North pole magnetic water. Apply a North pole magnet or wrist band to the Ney Guan point on the inner wrist about three finger widths above the crease between the arm and the hand.

Bites (insect)
Treat as quickly as possible using North pole energy. **See Bee Stings**

Bladder conditions
Apply North pole energy daily using a magnetic mattress pad or ceramic block magnets. Drink North pole water. Drink water from both poles if kidney stones are a factor.

Bladder irritable
PMF therapy is an optional treatment with this ailment.

Blepharitis (inflammation of the eye lid)
Apply small North pole magnets to the closed eyelids. Wash the eyes with North pole water.

Blood Circulation (poor)
A professional diagnosis is essential. Use magnetic therapy as a supplement to conventional treatment. To improve circulation apply bipolar magnetic pads or wraps. Use a North pole magnetic mattress pad. Turn it over to sleep on the South pole on alternate days.

Hands - fingers Use bipolar wrist bands, rings and wraps.
Neck - arms Use a magnetic necklace.
Ankles - feet Use bipolar magnetic insoles and wraps.
Total body Use a North pole magnet near the heart to oxygenate the blood. Do not use with a pacemaker. PMF therapy is an optional treatment to increase circulation.

Blood-pressure high (hypertension)
A professional diagnosis is essential.Use magnetic therapy as a supplement to conventional treatment. Alternative treatments include using a North pole mattress and pillow. Wear a North pole magnetic wrist band on the right wrist. Apply a North pole magnet over the heart area and to the right side of the neck. Drink North pole water.

Blood-pressure low (hypotension)
A professional diagnosis is essential. Use magnetic therapy as a supplement to conventional treatment. Wear a South or alternating pole magnetic wrist band on the left wrist. Drink water magnetized with both poles daily. Use an alternating pole magnetic mattress or rotate a North pole mattress using the South pole side on alternate days. Use a North pole magnetic pillow. PMF therapy is an option with this ailment.

Boils - See Abscess

Bowel (spastic)
Apply a North pole ceramic magnet to the lower abdomen. If discomfort persists consult a health care professional. Drink 6 to 8 glasses of water magnetized with both poles daily. PMF therapy is an excellent option with this ailment.

Brain allergies
Refer to Dr. W. Philpott's book, Brain Allergies, available at libraries and book stores.

Brain Circulation

PMF therapy is an optional treatment to increase circulation. A bipolar magnetic necklace can also be used. Sleep on a North pole magnetic pillow. Refer to Dr. William Philpott's book, Brain Allergies.

Breast (lumps)

A professional diagnosis is essential. Use magnetic therapy as a supplement to conventional treatment. Refer to Dr. William Philpott's book, Cancer, The Magnetic Oxygen Answer. Treatments include using North pole energy with ceramic, neodymium or flexible rubber magnets. The magnet must be larger in size than the lesion. Do not use magnets with a pacemaker. Drink North pole water daily.

Bright's Disease (Nephritis)

A professional diagnosis is essential. Use magnetic therapy as a supplement to conventional treatment. Alternative treatments include using a North pole magnetic mattress. Apply a North pole ceramic block to the kidney area. Drink water magnetized with both poles.

Bronchitis

Use the South pole of a magnetic block or strip. Begin cautiously as congestion may break up quickly and cause excessive coughing. Follow with north pole treatment over the lung and throat area. Do not use magnets with a pacemaker. PMF therapy is an option with this ailment.

Burns

Apply a North pole magnet immediately to arrest pain and inflammation. When inflammation and pain subside, apply South pole to stimulate the healing process. Cover the affected skin with clean gauze before applying the magnet.

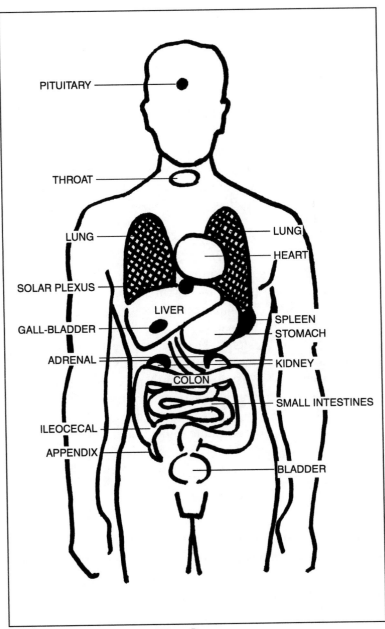

The Organs

65

Bruising
Use a flat ceramic magnet. Apply North pole for 2 or 3 days. When the bruise has stabilized, apply South pole energy to stimulate circulation.

Bursitis
Apply a North pole magnetic wrap or sleeve. A flexible bi-polar pad is effective where increased circulation is required.

Cancer
A professional diagnosis is imperative. Use magnetic therapy as a supplement to conventional treatment. Dr. William Philpott, Dr. Nevelle Bengali, and Dr. Goesta Wollin have affirmed the use of North pole magnetic energy to check tumor growth and cause size reduction. Specific treatment protocols using permanent magnets are outlined in Dr. William Philpott's literature. The choice of magnet will depend on the size of the tumor. The magnet must be larger than the lesion to eliminate the effect of South pole energy from the edges of the magnet. Neodymium magnets are preferred for small lesions. The South pole of a neodymium pendant worn over the thymus gland may stimulate the immune system. After using the South pole, rebalance using the North pole. Use a high strength North pole magnetic mattress or make a high strength magnetic bed by placing a series of North pole ceramic block magnets between the mattress and box spring. Placing the magnets 6 to 8 inches below the body eliminates the South pole effect between the magnets. Drink 6 to 8 glasses of North Pole water daily.

Candida
Sit on the North pole of a 4 x 6 x 1/2 inch ceramic magnet for 2 to 3 hours each day. Drink North pole magnetic water daily.

Carbuncle - See Abscess

Carpal Tunnel Syndrome
The North pole is recommended for pain, South pole for stimulation. The best compromise is a neodymium magnetic wrist band using both poles. In chronic conditions, a South pole band may be more beneficial.

Cataracts
Use North pole glasses that have small magnets attached to the temples. The magnets should be positioned on each side opposite the eye. Begin slowly and work up to an hour or two each day. Drink North pole water daily.

Cellulite deposits
Treat directly with North pole magnets. Use a north pole magnetic mattress and pillow. Drink North pole magnetic water.

Cervical Spine Syndrome
PMF therapy is an option with this ailment.

Cholesterol (high)
A professional diagnosis is important. Use magnetic therapy as a supplement to conventional treatment. Drink North pole magnetic water. Use a magnetic necklace to stimulate the thyroid area. Wear a North pole magnetic disk in the breast pocket or bra. Use a North pole magnetic mattress and pillow. Do not use magnets with a pacemaker.

Chronic Fatigue Syndrome - See Auto-immune disorders

Circulation - See Blood Circulation

Colitis (spastic)
Apply North pole energy using a ceramic block or rubber magnet. Apply several times a day for periods of 30 to 60 minutes. PMF therapy is an option with this ailment. Drink 6 to 8 glasses of North pole water daily.

Common Cold

Use a magnetic pendant on the thymus gland, to stimulate the immune system. Use South to stimulate then North to re-balance. Treat sinus areas with North pole magnetic strips or magnetic mask. Treat swollen glands with North pole magnets or a neck wrap. Drink North pole water daily.

Constipation

Apply the South pole of a ceramic block to the lower left abdomen for 30 minutes several times a day. Rebalance each time with 10 minutes of North pole energy. Drink 6 to 8 glasses of magnetic water daily. Drink South pole water initially and switch to both pole water when the condition is corrected. PMF therapy is a good option.

Cramp (muscular)

Apply South pole energy for 10 to 20 minutes to increase circulation then apply North pole energy to decrease pain and promote healing. PMF therapy is considered a good option with this ailment.

Cramps (menstrual)

Apply a bipolar magnetic pad to the lower abdomen to increase circulation and reduce pain.

Crohn's Disease - See Auto-immune disorders

Cystitis

Use the North pole of a ceramic block magnet or rubber magnet over the cyst for 1 to 3 hours daily. Sleep on a North pole magnetic mattress. Drink North pole water daily.

Dandruff

Magnetize shampoo with a North pole magnet. Rinse after shampooing with North pole water. Drink North pole water daily.

Deafness - See Ear Disease

Depression
Use a North pole magnetic mattress and pillow. Drink north pole water daily. PMF therapy is an option with this ailment. Place the device under the pillow while sleeping.

Dermatitis
Use a North pole magnetic mattress and pillow. Treat creams and ointments with the North pole of a ceramic magnet. If stress is a factor, (Psoriasis, Eczema) use a magnetic necklace. Drink 6 to 8 glasses of North pole water daily. Use North pole water when washing.

Detoxification
Sleep on a North pole magnetic mattress and pillow. Drink 6 to 8 glasses of North pole water daily.

Diabetes
A professional diagnosis is essential. Use magnetic therapy as a supplement to conventional treatment. Use alternating pole magnetic insoles and bracelets to improve circulation in the feet and hands. Sleep on a magnetic mattress and use a North pole magnetic pillow. Drink water magnetized with both poles. PMF therapy is an option with this ailment. **See Pancreas (underactive)**

Diarrhea
Apply North pole magnetic energy with a rubber strip or ceramic block magnet on the abdomen. Drink North pole magnetic water.

Disease prevention
A regular medical checkup is important. Use a North pole mattress and pillow for deep restorative sleep. Drink plenty of filtered magnetic water daily and exercise regularly. Eat primarily fruit, nuts, whole grains and vegetables. Get fresh

air and a moderate amount of natural sunlight daily. Use alcohol in moderation. Do not use tobacco.

Diverticulitis
Drink 6 to 8 glasses of both pole magnetic water daily. Apply a North pole magnet to the pain focus. To relieve constipation, apply a South pole magnet to the left abdomen for 15 to 30 minutes. Always rebalance with the North pole side. Use a North pole magnetic mattress.

Duodenal ulcer
Drink North pole magnetized milk and water daily. Sleep on a North pole magnetic mattress to relieve stress, and wear a magnetic necklace to relieve tension. PMF therapy is a possible option with this ailment. Follow the manufacturer's frequency suggestions.

Ear Disease
A professional diagnosis is essential. If caused by an infection, apply North pole energy with a small ceramic block magnet as an adjunct to conventional treatment.

Eczema - See Dermatitis

Edema (swelling)
A professional diagnosis is recommended. Apply North pole magnetic energy using a ceramic block or flexible pad. Drink both pole magnetic water.

Electromagnetic pollution
North pole energy is beneficial, as the creation of negative ions offsets positive ions produced by electromagnetic pollution. Use a North pole mattress and pillow. Drink North pole water daily. Wear a magnetic bracelet, pendant or necklace to balance the body during and after exposure.

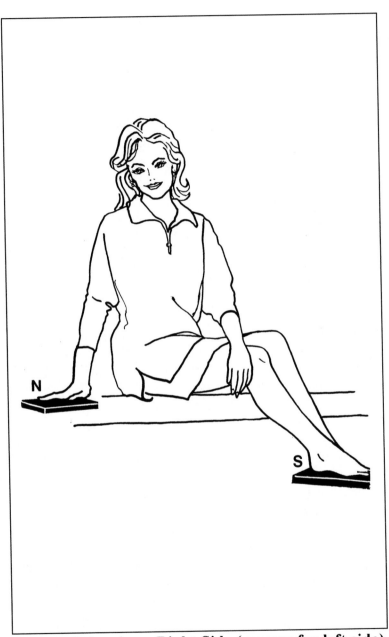

Energy Balancing - Right Side (reverse for left side)

Note: There is no evidence to substantiate the claim that permanent magnets worn on the body absorb or dissipate electromagnetic pollution.

Emotional Disorders
A professional diagnosis is essential. Use magnetic therapy as a supplement to conventional treatment. Refer to Dr. William Philpott's books, Brain Allergies and The Biomagnetic Handbook, where he describes various magnetic treatments.

Emphysema - See Asthma

Energy (low)
Sleep on a magnetic mattress. Rotate or turn the mattress every 2 or 3 days to use North pole then South pole. Repeat the cycle as long as required. An alternating pole mattress pad may also be used . **Note**: Most mattress pads made in North America utilize North pole on the top side. The magnetic field will extend at least 10 to 12 inches above the standard magnetic mattress and higher with high strength models. Do not use the South pole by itself for extended periods. Always rebalance with the North pole side. Drink both pole magnetic water daily.

Energy Balancing
If you are right handed, your right foot, hand and right side are South-positive, while your left hand, foot and side are North-negative. **Note**: About 10% of the population are left handed and may have the opposite polarity. They might try opposite suggestions to all of the following.

- For general treatment use ceramic block magnets. Apply North pole energy to the right hand and South pole energy to the left hand for 15 to 30 minutes. Repeat this process using the same polarity application on the feet.

- Ailments affecting the right side of the body: Using ceramic block magnets, apply North pole to the right hand and South pole to the right foot.
- Ailments affecting the left side of the body: Using ceramic block magnets, apply South pole to the left hand and North pole to the left foot.
- Ailments affecting the lower torso: Using ceramic block magnets, apply North pole to the right hand and South pole to the left foot.
- Ailments affecting the lower body including the legs: Using ceramic block magnets, apply North pole to the right foot and South pole to the left foot.
- Ailments affecting the upper body including the arms: Using ceramic block magnets, apply North pole to the right hand and South pole to the left hand.

Epilepsy
A professional diagnosis is essential. Use magnetic therapy as a supplement to conventional treatment. Use the North pole of a ceramic block magnet placed under the head between the mattress and box spring or possibly under the pillow. Begin with caution and close observation. Drink North pole magnetic water.

Eye Disease
A professional diagnosis is essential. Use magnetic therapy as a supplement to conventional treatment. Use North pole magnetic glasses. Wash eyes often with North pole magnetic water. **See Cataracts and Blepharitis**

Fatigue - See Energy (low) and/or Energy Balancing

Fever
Apply North pole using a small ceramic magnet, flexible disk or head band to the forehead. Apply a North pole magnet to the lower abdomen. Drink North pole water.

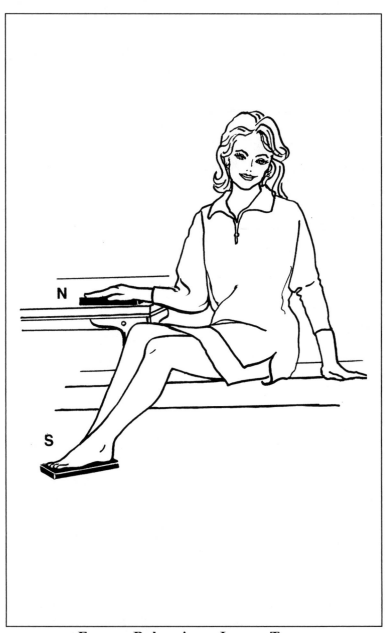

Energy Balancing - Lower Torso

Fibrositis - Fibromyalgia
Use a high strength North pole magnetic mattress or ceramic block sleep system. North pole energy may be applied to specific pain sites using magnets, magnetic body wraps or wrist bands. Drink North pole magnetic water daily.

Fibroid Tumors - See Breast Lumps

Flatulence
Apply the North pole of a magnetic disk or block to the lower abdomen. Drink magnetic water from both poles.

Food Addiction
Use small magnets or ear studs on the acupuncture points in the ear that relate to stress and weight control. **See Obesity**

Foot Pain
Wear bipolar magnetic insoles or shoe inserts. These may also be worn through the night inside a pair of socks. Magnetic expansion bands or magnetic wraps worn on the ankles are also beneficial.

Fracture
Apply North pole energy as quickly as possible to establish the healing polarity. If a cast is applied, a North Pole magnet may be taped directly over the fracture as the magnetic field will penetrate the cast. PMF therapy is a good option.

Fracture (non-union)
Place a North pole magnet over the fracture and South pole magnet below the fracture. This will create an energy flow across the fracture enabling healing to begin. PMF treatment may be also be applied. Small portable devices can be used several hours daily while larger clinical units can be used for shorter time periods. Use frequencies and time sequences specified in the manufacturer's treatment manuals.

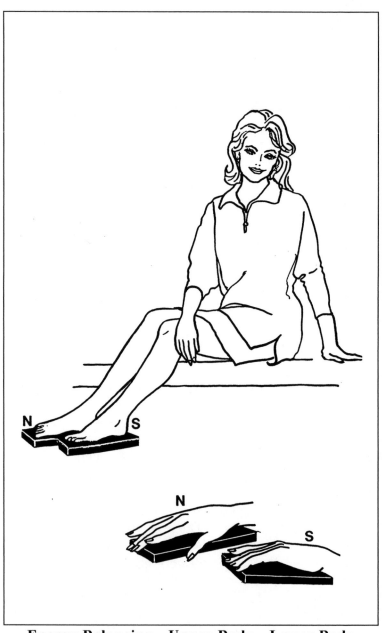

Energy Balancing - Upper Body - Lower Body

Frozen Shoulder

This should respond best using both poles alternately; North pole to sedate the pain and South pole to stimulate circulation. Apply alternating magnetic energy with either an alternating pole magnetic pad or PMF therapy.

Gallstones

A professional diagnosis is essential Use magnetic therapy as a supplement to conventional treatment. Apply the North pole magnet and drink both pole magnetic water.

Gastric Ulcer

Use a North pole magnet over the pain focus. Drink North pole magnetic water daily.

Gastritis

Alkalize with North pole energy using a ceramic block magnet applied to the abdomen. Do not apply within 60 to 90 minutes of eating. Drink North pole magnetic water.

Geomagnetic Disturbance

Researchers are discovering this to be a contributing factor in many disease conditions. The location should be checked by a qualified professional to determine the extent of the problem. Solutions may require moving the bed to a different location or to a different room. Position the head of the bed to the North if possible. Use a North pole magnetic mattress and pillow. A magnetic head board made with North pole ceramic block magnets is often helpful. Wear a magnetic bracelet, necklace or pendant. Drink North pole water daily.

Glaucoma - See Cataracts

Glandular Disease

A professional diagnosis is essential. Hyperactive conditions may be treated with North pole magnetic energy. Hypoactive conditions may be treated with South pole energy. Do not use the South pole if there is possibility of infection or malignancy. Always rebalance with North pole after using South pole energy.

Glands (Swollen)
A professional diagnosis is essential to determine the cause. Use magnetic therapy as a supplement to conventional treatment. Use North pole magnets to reduce infection and inflammation. Drink North pole magnetic water daily.
See Auto-immune disorders

Goiter (hyperthyroidism)
A professional diagnosis is essential. Use magnetic therapy as a supplement to conventional treatment. Apply North pole magnetic energy to the thyroid using a magnetic pendant or disk. Drink North pole water daily.

Gout
Alkalize the system using a North pole magnetic mattress and pillow. Drink 6 to 8 glasses of North pole water daily.

Hair Loss
Expose the scalp to the North pole using a flexible magnet. Massage the scalp using magnetized oil (both poles). This will also reduce dandruff. PMF therapy is an optional treatment with this ailment.

Hay Fever
PMF therapy is considered an optional treatment for this ailment. Follow the user's manual for frequency selections.

Hemorrhoids
Sit on the North pole of a ceramic block magnet for 1 hour, 2 to 3 times each day. Drink at least 6 glasses of North pole magnetic water daily. It is important to exercise daily, walking is recommended. PMF therapy is an option with this ailment.

Headache (new, acute)
A professional diagnosis is essential. Use magnetic therapy as a supplement to conventional treatment.

Headache (chronic)
Use a North pole magnetic head wrap. A magnetic necklace may be helpful for migraine. Drink North pole magnetic water daily. Use a North pole magnetic mattress if stress is a factor. PMF therapy is an option. Use a portable device over the sternum during the day and under the pillow at night.

Healing (wounds or sores)
Wash with North pole magnetic water. Use a North pole magnet, but do not apply directly. Cover the wound with a gauze bandage then apply the magnet. The magnet should be larger in area than the lesion being treated. When healing has begun, an alternating pole magnetic pad may be used.

Heart - See Angina, Arrhythmia and Arteriosclerosis

Heartburn (indigestion)
Place a North pole magnet over the pain focus to alleviate acidic conditions. Drink at least 6 glasses of North pole magnetic water daily.

Heel Spur
Wear bipolar magnetic insoles or shoe inserts.

Hernia
A professional diagnosis is recommended. North pole may be used to contract muscles in early stages. Drink North pole magnetic water.

Herniated Disk - See Back Pain

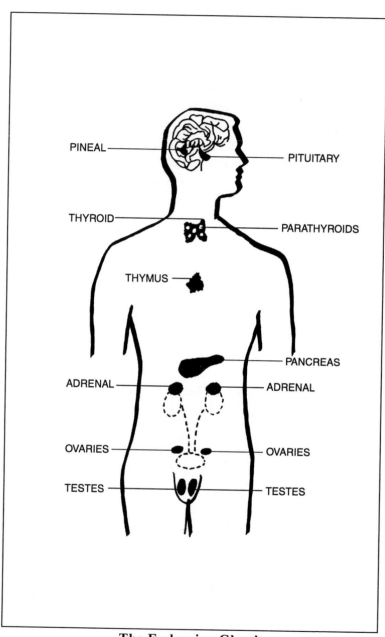

The Endocrine Glands

Hiccups
Place a North pole magnet over the breast bone. Drink North pole magnetic water. PMF therapy may be effective with this problem.

High Blood Pressure - See Blood Pressure (high)

Hodgkin's Disease - See Cancer

Hot Flashes - See Menopause

Hyperactivity
Use a North pole magnetic mattress and pillow. Drink North pole water daily. Wear a magnetic necklace if stress is a possible factor. PMF therapy is an option with this ailment. Place the applicator under the pillow at night.

Hypertension - See Blood pressure (high)

Hypotension - See Blood pressure (low)

Hyperthyroidism
Wear a North pole magnetic pendant. Use a North pole magetic pillow. Drink North pole magnetic water daily.

Hypothyroidism
Wear a bipolar necklace or pendant. Use a magnetic mattress. Rotate on a daily basis using the South pole side one day, the North pole side the next. Repeat as long as necessary. Drink South pole magnetic water. **See Glandular Disease**

Immune Deficiency - See Auto-immune disorders

Immunity Poor
Use a South pole or both pole pendant to stimulate the thymus gland. Rebalance with North pole if the South pole is

applied separately. PMF therapy is an option with this ailment.

Impotency
Sit on the South pole of a ceramic block magnet for 1 hour, 2 or 3 times a day. Follow each session with 10 minutes of North pole treatment. Repeat as long as required. Drink both pole magnetic water. **Note**: Do not use the South pole with inflammation, infection or malignancy. PMF therapy is an option with this ailment.

Indigestion - See Heartburn

Infection
Wash with North pole water. Apply a North pole magnet of an appropriate size to completely cover the lesion. Cover the area with a gauze bandage before applying any magnet. Drink North pole water daily.

Infection (Viral)
Use a North pole mattress and pillow. Drink North pole magnetic water daily.

Inflammation
Apply North pole energy with a ceramic or rubber magnet. Wash the area with North pole water. PMF therapy is an optional treatment using the specific frequency recommended by the manufacturer of the device.

Influenza
Use a North pole mattress and pillow. Drink North pole magnetic water daily. PMF therapy is an option with this ailment. Place the applicator under pillow while sleeping and over the sternum through the day.

Insomnia
Use a North pole magnetic pillow and mattress. Drink North pole magnetic water. PMF therapy is a good option. Place the applicator under the pillow while sleeping.

Irritable Bowel - See Bowel (spastic)

Jaundice - See Liver Disease

Jet Lag
Use a North pole magnetic pillow. PMF therapy is an option with this condition.

Joint Disease - See Arthritis

Keloid (scar tissue)
Use North pole or bipolar magnetic pads to diminish scar tissue.

Keratitis - See Cataracts

Knee Ailments
Wraps containing alternating pole magnets provide increased circulation and pain relief for chronic conditions. Painful knee problems resulting from athletic injuries may be treated with wraps, providing either North pole or alternating pole energy. North pole is recommended for new injuries.
Caution is necessary in treating athletic injuries because magnetic treatment will alleviate pain. This may encourage the injured person to return to normal activity before the injury is completely healed.

Kidney Stones
Professional diagnosis and treatment are essential. Consider magnetic therapy as a supplement to conventional treatment. Use a North pole ceramic block to reduce pain by placing

the magnet over the focus of the pain. Drink 6 to 8 glasses of both pole magnetic water daily.

Laryngitis
Apply the North pole of a small magnet to the larynx. Apply a North pole neck wrap. Gargle with North pole water.

Learning Disorders (A.D.D.)
Use a North pole mattress and pillow. Drink North pole magnetic water daily.

Leukemia - See Cancer

Leukoderma
Stimulate the area with a South pole or an alternating pole magnetic pad. Massage the area with oil magnetized with both poles. Treat the affected area by exposing it to electro-magnetic energy from sunlight regularly. Wear a magnetic necklace to stimulate the thyroid. Drink both pole magnetic water.

Liver Disease
Professional diagnosis and treatment are essential. Place a large North pole ceramic block over the liver area for 30 to 60 minutes, twice daily. Use a North pole mattress and pillow. Drink both pole magnetic water daily.

Lumbago - See Arthritis

Lupus
Professional diagnosis and treatment are essential. PMF therapy has been found effective in some cases but use as an optional treatment only. **See Auto-immune disorders**

Lymphoma - See Cancer

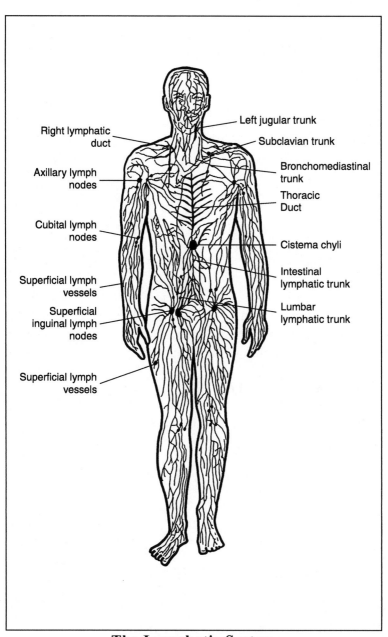

Right lymphatic duct

Axillary lymph nodes

Cubital lymph nodes

Superficial lymph vessels

Superficial inguinal lymph nodes

Superficial lymph vessels

Left jugular trunk

Subclavian trunk

Bronchomediastinal trunk

Thoracic Duct

Cistema chyli

Intestinal lymphatic trunk

Lumbar lymphatic trunk

The Lymphatic System

Lymphatic System

Stimulate the lymph system by walking or exercising regularly with a rebounder or mini-trampoline. Sleep on a high strength North pole mattress and pillow. Drink North pole magnetic water daily.

Magnetic Field Deficiency Syndrome

Use a high strength North pole mattress and pillow. Wear a magnetic wrist band, necklace or pendant or carry a small North pole magnet on the body. Drink water magnetized with both poles daily.

Mastoiditis

A professional diagnosis is essential. Apply North pole energy on the bone behind the ear using a small ceramic block magnet. A North pole head band is an alternative.

Memory (weak)

Use a North pole pillow at night and a North pole head band during the day. A magnetic necklace may benefit by stimulating circulation to the brain.

Melanoma - See Cancer

Meniere's Disease - See Ear Disease

Menopause

Use a North pole mattress and pillow. Drink North pole magnetic water daily.

Menses (suppressed) - See Amenorrhea

Menstrual Disorders

Apply a flexible bipolar magnetic pad to the lower abdomen. A flexible North pole magnet may also be effective. Drink North pole water daily.

Meningitis
Consider magnetic therapy as a supplement to conventional treatment. Use a high strength North pole mattress and pillow. Drink North pole magnetic water daily.

Mental Problems - See Emotional Disorders

Metatarsalgia
Use cushioned bipolar or North pole magnetic insoles.
See Foot Pain

Migraine
Use a North pole magnetic head band. A magnetic necklace may be of benefit if stress is a factor. PMF therapy is an option with this ailment. Use under the pillow at night and over the sternum during the day. **See Headache and Nausea**

Motion Sickness
Apply North pole energy to the inner wrist using a magnetic wrist band or small magnetic patch. A magnetic wrist band using alternating poles is also effective.

Multiple Sclerosis
A professional diagnosis is essential. Use magnetic therapy as a supplement to conventional treatment. Use a high strength North pole magnetic mattress and pillow. If North pole treatment does not help try using an alternating pole magnetic mattress. PMF therapy is an option with this ailment as it provides alternating magnetic fields. Follow the manufacturer's directions. **See Auto-immune disorders**

Muscle Spasm or Cramp
Apply South pole energy using a ceramic or rubber magnet to relax and soften contracted or strained muscles. Apply North pole energy to relieve pain and promote the healing process. An alternating pole magnetic pad can be used in place of the above combination.

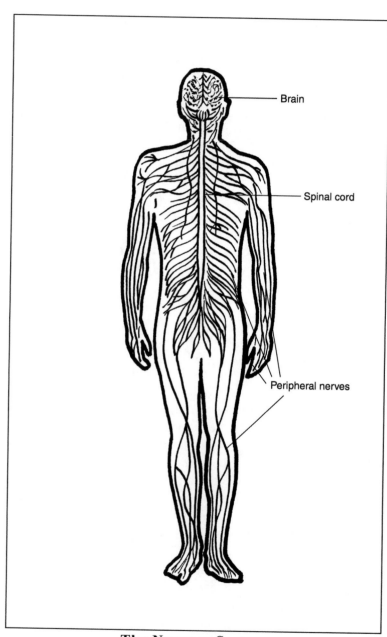

Brain

Spinal cord

Peripheral nerves

The Nervous System

Mumps
Apply North pole energy over the swelling. Drink North pole magnetic water.

Nausea
Apply North pole magnetic energy over the upper abdomen. Drink water magnetized with both poles. Wear a magnetic wrist band, to apply magnetic energy to the inner wrist 2 inches above the hand crease (Ney Guan, P6 acupuncture point). Do not use magnets during pregnancy.

Nephritis - See Bright's Disease

Neuralgia - Neuritis
Use a North pole mattress and pillow. Drink North pole magnetic water daily.

Nervous Tension
Use a North pole magnetic mattress and pillow. Wear a magnetic necklace to relieve tension in the shoulders. PMF therapy is an option with this ailment. Apply over the solar plexus during the day and under the pillow while sleeping.

Nicotine Addiction
Use small magnets or ear studs to treat acupuncture points in the ear relating to stress and nicotine withdrawal symptoms. Use a North pole magnetic mattress and pillow.

Numbness
A professional diagnosis is important. Use magnetic therapy as a supplement to conventional treatment. Wear a flexible alternating pole pad over the area. Wear alternating pole magnetic insoles for numbness in the feet. Use an alternating pole wrist band if numbness occurs in the hands and wrists. Drink water magnetized with both poles.

Obesity

The alkalinizing effect produced by North pole magnetic energy is considered effective in neutralizing and dissolving fat. Use a high strength magnetic mattress pad and pillow at night. During the day wear a North pole magnetic waist band or flexible magnet on the area to be treated. Drink at least 6 to 8 glasses of North pole magnetic water daily.
See Food Addiction

Orchitis (inflammation of testicle)

A professional diagnosis is important. Use magnetic therapy only as a supplement to conventional treatment. Sit on the North pole side of a ceramic block magnet for at least an hour, 2 or 3 times daily.

Osteo Arthritis - See Arthritis

Osteoporosis

Magnetic field deficiency may be a contributing factor. Use a high strength North pole magnetic mattress and pillow. Drink 6 to 8 glasses of North pole magnetic water daily. Use a pocket magnet, magnetic pendant, necklace or wrist band to supplement the Earth's natural magnetic field.
See Magnetic Field Deficiency Syndrome

Otis Media

Treat the infected area with magnetic energy by applying a North pole magnet. Wash with North pole water and drink North pole water daily. **See Ear Disease**

Ovarian Cysts - See Cystitis

Pain

Apply North pole energy using a ceramic or rubber magnet of the appropriate size. Use alternating pole wraps or pads when increased circulation is required, such as with muscle spasms or cramps. Magnetic wraps and appliances are available for all areas of the body. For complete body treatment use a North pole magnetic mattress and pillow. Drink 6 to 8 glasses of North pole water daily. PMF therapy is a good alternative.

Pancreas (underactive)
Magnetic therapy should be applied as a supplement to conventional treatment. Use the South pole of a ceramic block magnet. Place it over the pancreas for 30 minutes in the morning and evening. Rebalance with North pole energy for at least 10 minutes after using South pole treatment. For increased circulation in the feet wear bipolar magnet insoles. Drink both pole magnetic water.
See Diabetes

Pancreas (overactive)
Magnetic therapy should be applied only as a supplement to conventional treatment. Use a North pole magnetic mattress and pillow. Apply a North pole ceramic magnet over the pancreas for at least one hour each day. Drink North pole magnetic water.

Phlebitis
A professional diagnosis is important. Use magnetic therapy as a supplement to conventional treatment. Use a North pole magnetic pad or wrap. Drink both pole magnetic water.

Pleurisy
Use magnetic therapy as a supplement to conventional treatment. Apply North pole energy using a ceramic magnet. Drink 6 to 8 glasses of North pole water daily. If you use a pacemaker, do not use magnets.

PMS
Use a North pole magnetic mattress and pillow. A North pole magnetic headband may also be beneficial. Research indicates an alternating magnetic pad to be effective. Drink

both pole magnetic water daily. PMF therapy is a good option with this ailment.

Pneumonia
A professional diagnosis is important. Use magnetic therapy in conjunction with conventional treatment. Use a North pole magnetic pillow and mattress. Drink North pole water daily. If you use a pacemaker, do not use magnets.

Potency Impaired - See Impotency

Prolapsed Uterus
A professional diagnosis is important. Use magnetic therapy in conjunction with conventional treatment. Apply the South pole to the pubic area using a flexible magnetic strip for 1 hour twice daily. Rebalance with the North pole for 10 minutes after South pole application. Do not use the South pole if cyst, tumor or hemorrhoids are a factor.

Prostate Gland Disease
A professional diagnosis is important. Have a regular P.S.A. test. Magnetic therapy should be considered as a supplement to conventional treatment. Sit on the North pole of a ceramic magnet for several hours a day. Drink 6 to 8 glasses of North pole water daily. PMF therapy is an option with this ailment. See Glandular Disease

Psoriasis - See Dermatitis

Psychosomatic Illness
PMF therapy is an option with this ailment. Apply over the sternum during the day and under the pillow at night.

Raynaud's Disease
Magnetic therapy should be used as a supplement to conventional treatment. Use alternating pole wrist bands or ankle bands. Use bipolar magnetic insoles. Drink at least 6

to 8 glasses of water magnetized with both poles daily. PMF therapy is an option with this ailment.

Restless Leg Syndrome
Place an alternating pole magnetic pad between the knees while lying on one side. A magnetic leg wrap is also effective.

Rheumatoid Arthritis - See Arthritis (Rheumatoid)

Rheumatism - See Arthritis

Ringworm
Apply North pole magnetic energy using a flexible magnet. Wash the area with North pole water. Drink 6 to 8 glasses of North pole water daily.

Rotator Cuff Syndrome - See Frozen Shoulder

Ruptured Disk - See Back Pain

Sarcoma - See Cancer

Scar Tissue
Scars can be reduced and often removed with magnetic treatment. North pole and alternating pole treatments have produced good results. Use a North pole ceramic or flexible magnet or alternating pole magnetic pad. Apply daily for two to three months.

Sciatica
Use a North pole magnetic mattress and pillow. Wear a North pole magnetic back support or belt through the day. PMF therapy is an option. **See Back Pain**

Sea Sickness - See Motion Sickness

Shingles (Herpes Zoster)
A professional diagnosis is important. Use a North pole magnetic mattress and pillow. Magnetize creams and ointments with the North pole. Apply North pole directly to the rash with ceramic or rubber magnets. Drink 6 to 8 glasses of North pole water daily.

Sinusitis
Treat the area using a North pole mask, ceramic disks or rubber strips. Apply for 2 hours daily. Use a North pole magnetic pillow. Drink North pole magnetic water. PMF therapy is optional with this ailment.

Skin Conditions
Using a North pole magnetic mask will help offset the effect of aging skin and wrinkles. Drink both pole magnetic water. **See Acne and Dermatitis**

Sleep Problems - See Insomnia

Smoking (to stop) - See Nicotine Addiction

Snoring
Use a North pole magnetic pillow.

Sore Throat
Apply North pole magnetic energy to the affected area. A magnetic headband may be used under the chin or around the neck. Gargle several times a day with North pole water. Use a North pole mattress and pillow.

Sprains
Apply North pole or alternating pole magnetic strips or pads using an elastic bandage or brace. When healing has started use an bipolar magnetic pad to increase circulation.

Stomach Ulcers - See Ulcers

Stress - See Nervous Tension

Stroke
Professional attention is essential. Use magnetic therapy as a supplement to conventional treatment. Use a North pole magnet on the forehead and spine. If paralysis affects one side of the body only, apply North pole to the opposite side of the head. If speech is affected, apply North pole to the left side of the head. Care should be taken when applying a strong magnet to the head. For weakness on either side of the body follow the suggestions listed under **Energy Balancing**. Drink North pole water daily.

Synovitis
Use a North pole wrap or sleeve wrap on the joint for 6 to 8 hours a day. Drink North pole water daily.

Tendinitis
Treat the inflammation with North pole energy using an appropriate wrap or magnet. When the pain has subsided, apply a bipolar flexible pad to rejuvenate the tissue while providing pain relief. PMF therapy is a good option with this ailment.

Tennis Elbow - See Tendinitis

Thyroid Gland - See Glandular Disease

Tinnitis
A professional diagnosis is important. Magnetic treatment should be applied as a supplement to conventional therapy. Lack of circulation requires South pole or both pole application. Apply behind the ear using a small ceramic disk or flexible magnet. A magnetic head wrap may be suitable. Do not use strong magnets in this area. If the problem is the result of infection, use North pole application.

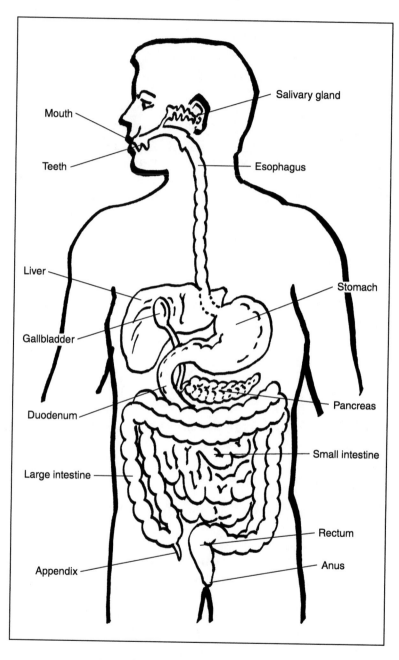

The Gastrointestinal System

Tonsillitis
Apply a North pole magnetic neck wrap. Drink North pole water daily. Gargle with North pole water.

Travel Sickness - See Motion Sickness

Tumor - See Cancer

Ulcers (Stomach)
Professional advice is important. Magnetic therapy should be applied as a supplement to conventional treatment. Use a North pole ceramic magnet on the pain focus. Do not use until one hour after eating. Drink 6 to 8 glasses of North pole water daily.

Ulcers (Skin)
Skin ulcers may be treated with an alternating pole pad. Apply over a gauze bandage. PMF therapy is an excellent optional treatment for this ailment.

Ulcers (Mouth)
Use a North pole mattress and pillow. Drink 6 to 8 glasses of North pole water daily. Gargle with North pole water.

Urinary Tract Conditions
Professional advice is essential. Magnetic therapy should be applied as a supplement to conventional treatment. Apply a North pole ceramic magnet over the kidneys. Drink 6 to 8 glasses of North pole water daily. If kidney stones are a possible factor, use water magnetized with both poles.

Vaginal Infection
Professional diagnosis is necessary. Use magnetic therapy as a supplement to conventional treatment. Sit on the North pole side of a ceramic magnet for 1 to 2 hours, 2 to 3 times a day. Drink North pole water daily.

Varicose Veins - See Phlebitis

Vertigo - See Ear Diseases

Warts
Apply a small North pole neodymium magnet. Homeopathic remedies are helpful both topically and internally.

Weight Control - See Food Addiction and Obesity

Writer's Cramp
Use a North pole magnetic mattress and pillow. Wear a magnetic necklace or wrist band to alleviate the stress associated with this condition.

Chapter 11

Related Therapies

Acupuncture and Magnetic Therapy

Acupuncture therapy and auricular therapy (ear acupuncture) used for centuries in China, is gaining popularity in many other parts of the world including Canada and the USA. Acupuncture is a healing art which has several variations including substituting magnets for the traditional needles. It requires special training to locate and use magnetic acupuncture, as the treatment points are not always located near the problem being treated. For example, to treat motion sickness or infection of the left inner ear, one stimulates the Ney Guan point which is located on the left inner wrist.

Small magnettys are useful as treatment for stress and muscular tension. The exact point location is not as important in this case. The magnets provide sufficient stimulation to soften and relax the tight muscles causing the problem.

There are many good books available on traditional acupuncture that enable the therapist to learn procedures and the treatment points. Small electronic detectors enable the novice therapist to locate the exact acupuncture point.

A book dealing specifically with magnetic acupuncture is <u>Magnetic Healing and Treatments</u>, by Noel Norris, a practitioner from Australia. Another good book in this field is <u>Magnet Therapy</u>, by Holger Hannemann, which also includes a useful section on the application of flexible alternating pole magnetic pads.

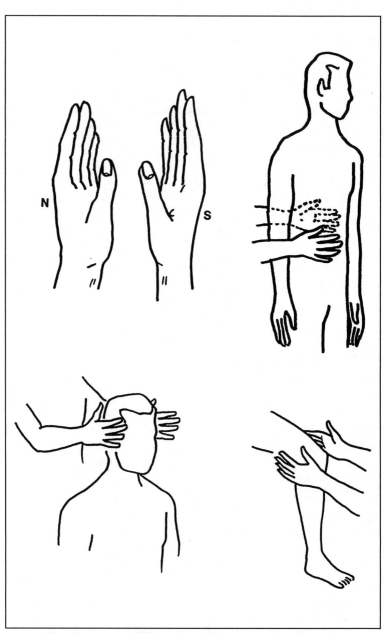

Laying on of Hands - Therapeutic Touch

Laying on of Hands - Therapeutic Touch

The use of this type of magnetic energy therapy is becoming widespread because Dolores Kreiger's book, Therapeutic Touch, has had a major impact on mainstream medicine. According to Professor Kreiger, therapeutic touch is a modern interpretation of several ancient healing methods. It is estimated that this method has been taught to over 35,000 doctors, nurses and health practitioners and is now taught in many American colleges.

Therapeutic touch does not necessarily require the practitioner to touch the body, though this is recommended for a few specific problems. Practitioners are trained to use their hands to feel the magnetic energy field of the patient. They can detect increases and decreases, allowing them to sense and treat problems by manipulating the patient's energy flow.

In addition to Dr. Kreiger's excellent book, two others can be recommended; Magnetic Therapy, by Abbot George Burke and The Rainbow In Your Hands, by Davis and Rawls.

Colour and Light Therapy

Sunlight is composed of a variety of energies that are transmitted to the earth as electromagnetic waves. About 1% of the overall electromagnetic spectrum is visible to the human eye. This 1% contains all the colours of the rainbow with violet being the shortest and red the longest visible wave length.

Ancient Egyptians were the first to use colour for healing and the Greeks were the first to document the theory and practice of solar therapy, as it was called. The Greek city of Heliopolis was noted for its healing temples where sunlight was broken up into the various colours and each colour was used as a specific therapy.

Magnetic journals from India outline the technique of treating water and liquids with traditional magnetic energy but also describe wrapping the containers in specific coloured paper and exposing them to sunlight. This enhances the liquid with the benefit of specific colour energy.

Modern medicine recognizes that light deprivation is the primary cause of S.A.D., a seasonal disorder produced by the reduced exposure to sunlight on short winter days and overcast conditions, common in the Northern hemisphere. It can be successfully treated with sunlight or full spectrum lighting. Other conditions which are commonly treated with light therapy are jaundice, bulimia, problematic sleep cycles and irregular menstrual cycles.

Light therapy is receiving increased attention and study. Colour Medicine, by Charles Klotsche, is an excellent book on the subject which outlines colour medicine schedules for over 123 specific disorders. Jacob Liberman's, Light, Medicine of The Future, is another excellent source of information.

As a result of photobiologist, John Ott's research, several important methods were developed utilizing light therapy with full-spectrum lighting. Several systems of colour therapy are available using specific colour slides and filters. The Dinshaw Health Society of New Jersey is a good source of information on this subject.

The newest equipment for this purpose combines advantages of colour therapy with the added benefits of specific pulsed frequencies that have been established in PMF therapy.

CHAPTER 12

Magnetic Water

Many experts, including Dr. William Philpott, Dr. Neville Bengalli, Dr. Albert Roy Davis, Walter Rawls, Dr. R. Broeringmeyer and Dr. F. K. Bellokossy have described the benefits of magnetic water.

Magnetizing water transforms it into a special liquid. In many countries magnetic water is used as a basic type of medication in conjunction with magnetic treatment.

It should be noted that three types of magnetic water and liquids are possible, each offering a different function:

Magnetic North pole water or liquids are used to wash and disinfect external lesions. They are used internally to promote an antacid, alkaline condition in the body and in treatments for bacterial, viral and parasitic infections.

Both pole magnetic water or liquids are used where a balance is needed. This is a general type of magnetic water, used by healthy individuals to revitalize their magnetic potential. It is also recommended in place of North pole water for those with kidney stone problems.

Magnetic South pole water and liquids are used internally when the body is depressed, tired and exhausted. Do not use when an infection or inflammation of any type is evident. South pole treatment will increase the effectiveness of massage oils.

What Magnetized Water Can Do
North pole magnetized water can help in the treatment of almost all diseases. Magnetic water has lower surface

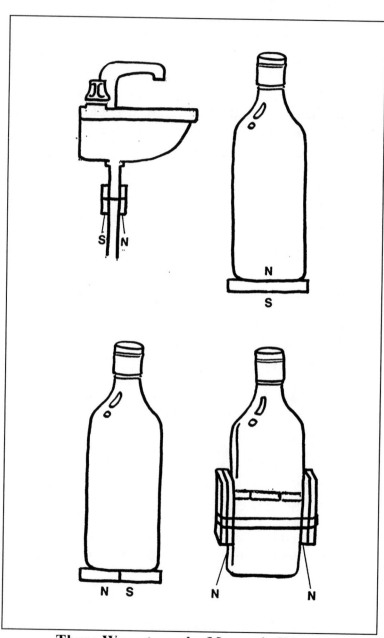

Three Ways to make Magnetic Water

tension which makes it more penetrating and more easily absorbed by the cells. It is beneficial in digestive disorders because it aids in the reduction of excess acid and bile in the digestive system and helps regulate bowel movement. Thus it improves digestion, increases appetite and imparts health and energy to the person who drinks it regularly. Many healthy people drink magnetized water daily to eliminate possible digestive disorders.

North pole water or liquids, such as fresh fruit juices may also benefit nervous disorders and blood pressure problems, especially low blood pressure. It offers a soothing and slightly sedative effect to the nervous system. Additional benefits are claimed by Russian doctors who utilize North pole treated water in clearing clogged arteries and normalizing the circulatory system. In addition North pole water is recommended as an aid in treating asthma, bronchitis, colds, coughs and fevers.

Magnetized water can also be used externally for washing sore or swollen eyes, wounds, and eczema spots. For eye infections, it is beneficial if the eyes are washed or sprayed with North pole water several times a day. Many references to magnetic water are outlined in **Chapter 10**, which deals with magnetic treatment for various ailments. North pole water is most often recommended. A general recommendation is to drink 6 to 8 glasses of magnetic water daily.

The reduced surface tension of magnetic water increases the the foaming action of soap. Cleaner skin, dishes and clothes are the result.

How to Make Magnetic Water

Magnetic water or liquids can be made in several ways. Water can be magnetized as it moves through the water pipe or by applying a magnet to a container of liquid.

Regular users of magnetic water keep a container of water or juice on a flat ceramic block magnet in the refrigerator. If water is treated while moving through the pipe it will be fully magnetized as it comes out of the tap. If a large container of still water is treated with magnets it will require several hours to become fully magnetized.

Three ways to make North pole water

1. Attach a North pole magnet or a set of North pole magnetic clamps on either side of the cold water pipe. This method works on copper, plastic or stainless steel pipe.

2. Place a container of water or liquid on the North pole face of a flat magnet. The magnet should be at least 4" x 6" x 1/2" thick. The container can be made of glass, plastic, stainless steel or copper.

3. Tape the North pole side of two ceramic magnets, which are at least 2" x 5" x 1/2" in size, on opposite sides of the container.

Three ways to make both pole water

1. Attach a North pole magnet on one side and the South pole of a magnet on the other side of the cold water pipe close to the tap. This method will work on pipes made of copper, plastic or stainless steel.

2. Tape the North pole side of a ceramic magnet (at least 2" x 5" x 1/2" in size) to one side and a South pole magnet on the other side of a container made from glass, plastic, stainless steel or copper.

3. Place a container of water or liquid over the juncture of two ceramic block magnets which have been placed together,

one magnet with the North side up and the other with South side up.

Three ways to make South pole water

1. Attach a South pole magnet or a set of South pole magnetic clamps on either side of the cold water pipe. This method works on copper, plastic or stainless steel pipe.

2. Place a container of water or liquid on the South pole face of a flat magnet. The magnet should be at least 4" x 6" x 1/2" thick. The container can be made of glass, plastic, stainless steel or copper.

3. Tape the South pole sides of 2 ceramic magnets at least 2" x 5" x 1/2" in size on opposite sides of a container made of glass, plastic, stainless steel or copper.

Prove it to Yourself

An interesting test can be performed with dry or bitter wine, black coffee or unsweetened grapefruit juice. Use three small containers and two magnets. Mark the containers 1, 2 and 3, placing container #1 on a North pole magnet, #2 on a South pole magnet, and leave #3 as the control unit. Fill all containers with the liquid, let sit for 30 to 60 minutes, and then do a taste test. You will find that the South pole liquid will taste smooth and sweet and the North pole liquid will taste tart and sharp. The control liquid will not change, of course. South pole treatment causes an acidic reaction which mellows a sharp bitter tasting liquid. North pole treatment causes an alkaline reaction that will increase the sharp bitter taste of the original liquid.

Other Uses of Magnetic Water

Scale Control
Magnetizing a water system provides an alternative to chemical treatment where large amounts of minerals are present in the water. Hard water scale in pipes and appliances is usually controlled with costly chemical treatments that often create pollution. Magnetizing a water system is inexpensive and maintenance free. It is used to treat water in homes and commercial buildings and has many uses in industry such as controlling the scale build up in boilers and cooling towers.

Agriculture
Magnetic water has a positive effect on plant growth. Magnetized water is more solvent and more readily absorbed because of its lower surface tension. This increases absorption of the dissolved nutrients in the water. Studies carried out in conjunction with the Israeli Institute of Technology in Haifa indicated that the use of magnetized irrigation water on plants resulted in:
- Greater uniformity in the growth and vitality of the crops
- A reduction in fertilizer use
- Reduction of mineral build-up in pipes and spray heads
- Longer producing season
- Improved quality of size, shape, sugar level, and leaves
- 13% to 20% increase in production

Magnetized water has proven beneficial when given to animals. Tests conducted in Israel recorded the following:
- Reduced mortality, better health and more vitality
- Increased weight of cattle, calves, sheep and fowl
- Dairy cattle and hens had longer production seasons
- Reduction of feed quantities was possible
- The reduction of algae, lime deposits and other foreign elements improved the quality of the drinking water

Bibliography

- Bhattacharya Dr. A.K., Healing By Magnets
- Bhattacharya Dr. A.K., Power of Magnets
- Bhattacharya Dr. A.K. and Dr. R.U. Sierra, Power of a Magnet to Heal
- Bhattacharya Dr. A.K., The Magnetic Study of Life
- Bansal, Dr. H.L. and Dr. R.S., Magnetic Cure for Common Diseases
- Bansal, Dr. H. L., Magneto Therapy
- Barnothy, Dr. Madeline F., Biological Effects of Magnetic Fields
- Becker, Dr. R.O. and Gary Seldon, The Body Electric
- Becker, Dr. R.O., Cross Currents
- Bengali, Dr. Nevelle S., Magnet Therapy Theory and Practice
- Boericke, Dr. W., Homeopathic Materia Medica
- Broeringmeyer, Dr. R., Bio Health Enterprises, Bioenergy Newsletters
- Broeringmeyer, Dr. R. & Dr. Mary Broeringmeyer, Bio Health Enterprises, Energy Therapy Training Manual
- Broeringmeyer, R Dr., Principals of Magnetic Therapy
- Burke, Abbot George, Magnetic Therapy - Healing Power in Your Hands
- Coghill Research Laboratories, Gwent GB: Proceedings of the First World Congress in Magnetotherapy, 1996
- Davis Dr. A.R., The Anatomy of Biomagnetism
- Davis Dr. A.R., and W.Rawls, Magnetism & Its Effect on the Living System
- Davis Dr. A.R., and W.Rawls, The Magnetic Blueprint of Life
- Davis Dr. A.R., and W.Rawls, The Magnetic Effect
- Davis Dr. A.R., and W.Rawls, The Rainbow In Your Hands
- Davis Dr. A.R. and Dr. A.K. Bhattacharya, Magnet and Magnetic Fields

- Dinshah, Darius, <u>Spectro-Chrome Metry Encyclopaedia</u>
- Dinshah, Darius, <u>Let There be Light</u>
- <u>Encyclopaedia Britannica</u>, 15th Edition, Vol.15, <u>The</u> theoretical significance of left and right electron spin in the human energy system
- Fink, John M., <u>Third Opinion</u>, Magnet Therapy P27, 65, 92, 104,106
- Gerber, Dr. Richard, <u>Vibrational Medicine</u>, various references
- Goldberg Burton, <u>Alternative Medicine</u>, Magnetic Field Therapy, P 330
- Gordon, Barbara, <u>Medical Magnets</u>
- Hallett, Dr. Mark and Dr. Leonardo G. Cohen, <u>Magnetism, A New Method for Stimulation of Nerve and Brain</u>. JAMA, July 1989
- Hannemann, Holger, <u>Magnet Therapy, Balancing Your Body's Energy Flow</u>
- Heimlich, Jane, <u>What Your Doctor Won't Tell You</u>, Energy Medicine
- Holzapfel, Dr. E. P. Crepon and C. Philippe, <u>Magnet Therapy</u>
- Hoyer, Wulf D. <u>Geheilt Durch Magnetismus</u>. (German Language)
- Klotsche Charles, <u>Color Medicine</u>, secrets of color and vibrational healing
- Kreiger, Dolores Ph.D. R.N., <u>Accepting Your Power to Heal</u>
- Kreiger, Dolores Ph.D. R.N., <u>The Therapeutic Touch</u>
- Kokoschinegg, Dr. Peter and Dr. Gerald Fischer, <u>Effects of Pulsed Magnetic Fields on Biological Systems</u>, Magnets, April/ 1988.
- Kokoschinegg, Dr. Peter, <u>The Effects of Alternating Magnetic Fields in Medicine</u>, Magnets in Your Future, April 1991

- Kokoschinegg, Dr. Peter, <u>Magnetic Foils and their Application in Human Medicine</u>, Magnets in Your Future, April 1992
- Krohn Dr. Jacqueline, Frances Taylor and Jinger Prosser, <u>Natural Detoxification</u>
- Liberman, Dr. Jacob, Light, <u>Medicine of the Future</u>
- MacIvor, Virginia and Sandra LaForest, <u>Vibrations - Healing through Color etc.</u>
- Media, Dr. A.K., <u>Magnet Therapy and Acupuncture</u>
- Moss, Ralph W. Ph.D., <u>Cancer Therapy</u>, various references
- Nakagawa Dr. Kyoichi, <u>Magnetic Field Deficiency Syndrome and Magnetic Treatment</u>, Japan Medical Journal 2745, December 1976
- National Geographic, Vol.171, No.1, January 1987, <u>Medicine's New Vision</u>
- Norris, Noel C., <u>The Book of Magnetic Healing and Treatments</u>
- Ott, John N., <u>Health and Light</u>
- Payne, Dr. Buryl, <u>The Body Magnetic</u>
- Payne, Dr. Buryl, <u>Getting Started in Magnetic Therapy</u>
- Philpott, Dr. William H., and Sharon Taplin, <u>The Bio-magnetic Handbook</u>
- Philpott, Dr. William H., Cancer, <u>The Magnetic Oxygen Answer</u>
- Philpott, Dr. William H., <u>Brain Allergies</u>
- Pittman, U.L., Magnetism and Plant Growth., <u>Canadian Journal of Plant Science</u>
- Shepard, Dr. Stephan Paul, <u>Healing Energies</u>
- Swantani, M.T., <u>The Art of Magnetic Healing</u>
- Swantani, M.T., <u>Magnetotherapy for Common Diseases</u>
- Trock, Dr. David H. Dr. Alfred J. Bollet and Dr. Richard Markoll, <u>The Effect of Electromagnetic Fields in the Treatment of Osteoarthritis of the Knee and Cervical Spine, Journal of Rheumatology</u> October 1994

- Trexler, Gary, <u>The World of Light, Color, Health and Behavior</u>
- Walters, Richard, <u>Options,</u> The Alternative Cancer Therapy Book
- Washnis, George J. and Richard Z. Hricak, <u>Discovery of Magnetic Health</u>
- Wiancko. Dr. Ken, <u>Magnetotherapy, Ancient Wisdom, Modern Use,</u> Health Naturally April 1995
- Wollin, Dr. Goesta and Eric Enby, <u>Curing Cancer with Super Magnets</u>, Magnets in Your Future, April 1988
- World Health Organization, <u>Environmental Health Criteria</u>, Magnetic Fields 69
- Zimmerman, John, Ph.D., <u>Journals of the Bio-Electro-Magnetics Institute</u>

Illustrations

INDEX